CBS

Quick Text Revision Series
Important Text for Viva/MCQ's

OPHTHALMOLOGY

(For MBBS, BDS & Other Exams)

Second Edition

Editor

Dr. M.S. Bhatia

M.D., F.I.P., Dip. W.P.A., M.N.A.M.S.
Prof. & Head, Department of Psychiatry,
University College of Medical Sciences &
Guru Teg Bahadur Hospital,
Dilshad Garden, Delhi - 110 095 (India)

Contributing Editor

Dr. (Mrs.) Nirmaljit Kaur M.D.
Senior Specialist, Department of Microbiology,
Dr. R.M.L. Hospital,
New Delhi - 110 001 (India)

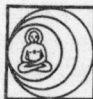

CBS

CBS PUBLISHERS & DISTRIBUTORS PVT. LTD.
New Delhi • Bengaluru • Pune • Kochi • Chennai

> ## Dedicated to
> ## Respected Teachers &
> ## Beloved Students

ISBN : 978-81-239-2025-2

First Edition : 2008
Second Edition : 2011

Published by Satish Kumar Jain and produced by V.K. Jain for
CBS Publishers & Distributors Pvt. Ltd.,
CBS Plaza, 4819/XI Prahlad Street, 24 Ansari Road, Daryaganj,
New Delhi - 110002, India.   • Website: www.cbspd.com
e-mail: delhi@cbspd.com, cbspubs@vsnl.com, cbspubs@airtelmail.in
Ph.: 23289259, 23266861, 23266867   • Fax: 011-23243014

Branches:
• *Bengaluru:* Seema House, 2975, 17th Cross, K.R. Road,
  Bansankari 2nd Stage, Bengaluru - 560070   Ph.: +91-80-26771678/79
  Fax: +91-80-26771680   • E-mail: cbsbng@gmail.com,
  bangalore@cbspd.com
• *Pune:* Bhuruk Prestige, Sr. No. 52/12/2+1+3/2,
  Narhe, Haveli (Near Katraj-Dehu Road By-pass), Pune - 411051
  Ph.: +91-20-64704058/59, 32342277 . • E-mail: pune@cbspd.com
• *Kochi:* 36/14, Kalluvilakam, Lissie Hospital Road,
  Kochi - 682018, Kerala • Ph.: +91-484-4059061-65
  Fax: +91-484-4059065   • E-mail: cochin@cbspd.com
• *Chennai:* 20, West Park Road, Shenoy Nagar, Chennai - 600030
  Ph.: +91-44-26260666, 26208620   • Fax: +91-44-42032115
  E-mail: chennai@cbspd.com

Printed at :
J.S. Offset Printers, Delhi

PREFACE TO THE SECOND EDITION

Medical science is a rapidly advancing field. Its new allied branches are coming up. In a competitive examination, more and more emphasis is being laid on these allied disciplines. But most of the standard textbooks of Ophthalmology have failed to devote adequate space to these new disciplines.

This New Quick Text Revision Series has been written with the aim to outline the major areas of various subjects.

Ophthalmology includes Factual Data, Important Points for Viva/MCQ's, Embryology, Commonest in Ophthalmology, Examination, Optics, Conjunctiva, Cornea and Sclera, Chambers, Uveal Tract, Lens, Glaucoma, Retina, Optic Nerve, Strabismus, Eye Lids, Names signs, syndrome & Tests & Miscellaneous,

This book will also be useul for MBBS, BDS and other Entrance Examinations

All suggestions for the modification of this book are welcome and will be duly acknowledged.

—Editors

CONTENTS

FACTUAL DATA ONE MUST KNOW

* Iron consists of prostaglandins E and F and causes breakdown of the tight junctions in the nonpigmented epithelium.

* Owing to its nutritional function, aqueous glucose concentration is 80% of that of plasma.

* The protein content of the aqueous is **1/90th** that of plasma.

* Uveoscleral outflow is approximately **0.3 ml/min** and is surprisingly independent of intraocular pressure changes. Aqueous production will remain constant until intraocular pressures are raised to **50 mmHg** and over.

* There is little difference between males and females until the age of 40, when the intraocular pressures becomes generally higher in woman.

* Accommodation is the **slowest** reaction of the triad, taking between **0.56s (near to far) and 0.64s.**

* Accommodation begins to develop at the age of **2 months** and is well developed by the **eighth month** of life. The accommodative power of a 2 years this has decreased to 10 diopters, and at 60 years of age, accommodation is no longer possible.

* The vitreous is a hydro sol-gel structure weighing approximately **3.9 g** and with a volume of **3.9 ml.**

* The pupil is capable of changing its diameter from **2 to 9 mm** (an 87% change).

* The superior rectus causes elevation (which is maximal if the eye is abducted **24°**), and in cyclotorsion (which is maximal on adduction or medial gaze). The inferior rectus causes depression (which is maximal in **24°** of abduction) and excyclotorsion (which is maximal in adduction).

* Smooth pursuit movements are designed to keep an object of interest on the fovea. They have a velocity of up to **100° per second** a latency of **125 ms.**

* Fixation movements are designed to move the retinal image by very small distances at regular intervals and prevent the image fading due to persistent bleaching of photoreceptor pigments (**Troxler's phenomenon**) more can have a frequency of up to **80Hz** and have an amplitude of **10-30°** of arc.

* Only **0.01%** of the body's total vitamin A is stored in the retina, the main store being the liver.

* Rod outer segment turnover time is approximately **9-13 days.**

* The proportion of blue cones relative to the other cones rises from 0 at the central 20° (where blue cones are totally absent) to a maximum at **7-10°.**

* Acuity in babies is determined by the techniques of preferential looking or measuring evoked potentials, in the newborn stripes (gratings) of about **1 cycle/degree** are the maximum resolvable that is **one thirtieth** of the adult level. Apart from the immature optical pathways, the neural connection of the retina and the visual cortex are not fully developed, and continue to differentiate until at least **8** years of age.

* The distance from the back of the globe to the optic foramen is **18 mm.**

* The following principles should be adhered to in orbital decompression in dysthyroid eye disease; lateral wall decompression achieves **2 mm** of retroplacement, orbital decompression may achieve up to **8 mm** of retroplacement, two-wall decompression is the **most commonly** used type.

* In blow out fractures of the orbit : enophthalmous may start **2 weeks** after the injury and progress up to **6 months,** diplopia is present in up-gaze and down-gaze. Water's view may detect an orbital floor fracture.

* Canaliculodacryocystorhinostomy (CDCR) is performed in lateral end common canalicular obstruction with **7 mm** of healthy canaliculus.

* A central corneal thickness of **0.6 mm** by pachometry is suggestive of endothelial dysfunction.

* Sarcoidosis shows uptake of **gallium 67** by mitotically active liposomes of granulocytes.

* In retinal photocoagulation: Argon laser emits coherent light of about **400 nm.** Xenon arc emits white light in the **350-1600 mm** range, the smaller the spot size of the laser, the greater the energy released.

* In **diabetic retinopathy:** Microaneurysms vary in size from **20 to 200 nm.** Microaneurysms are the **first clinically detectable signs,** hard exudates are located in the inner nuclear layer, macular oedema is the **most common** cause of visual impairment in background disease.

* In central retinal artery occlusion, one in five cases have preserved central vision due to a ciloretinal artery, slugging of the blood column is visible in both the arterioles and venules, the cherry red spot disappears in a few weeks, treatment should be initiated in all patients who present within **48 hours.**

* In the clinical evaluation of macula disease : **A x 16** slit lamp eye-piece may be used.

* In fluorescein angiography : 70-80% of fluorescein molecules are protein bound, the recirculation phase occurs within **three to five minutes.**

* The orbital axis forms an angle of **23 degrees** with the medial wall, the optic axis forms an angle of **23 degrees** with the orbital axis, the superior rectus is inserted at an angle of **23 degress** with the optical axis.

* The canaliculi are L-shaped structures with a short (**2 mm**) vertical portion and a longer (**10 mm**) horizontal portion. They normally unit to form a common canaliculus, which lies behind the medial palpebral ligament and pierces the lacrimal sac **2.5 mm** below its apex.

* In the normal adult, the levator is able to raise the upper lid by approximately **15 mm.**

* The superior fornix is situated **10 mm** from the limbus and the inferior **8 mm** from the limbus. The lateral fornix extends **14 mm** from the limbus.

* Corneal development begins at **day 33** of gestation.

* The cornea measures **1.1 mm** at the limbus and thins to **0.5 mm** centrally.

* Schwalbe's line marks the end of Descemet's membrane.

* Normal iris development is dependent on the closure of the embryonic fissure which occurs on **days 33-35.**

* The **collarette,** which lies approximately **2 mm** from the pupil margin, is the **thickest** region of the iris and divides it into a pupillary and ciliary zone.

* The lens is formed from a disc shaped thickening of the surface ectoderm overlying the optic vesicle on **day 27** of development.

* By **3 months** gestation the optic nerve is reached and by **5 months** the scleral spur is fully formed.

* **Bruch's membrane** is the innermost layer of the choroid and is approximately **2-4 mm** in thickness. It is five-layered structure.

* Sclera is thickest (**1 mm**) at its posterior pole, thins to **0.6 mm** at the equator and is thinnest (**0.3 mm**) immediately posterior to the tendinous insertions of the recti. The sclera is perforated **3 mm** medial and **1 mm** above the posterior pole by the optic nerve.

* Lamination is essentially completed by **4 months** and the ora serrata by **6 months.**

* The retina contains approximately **120 million** rods. They are **absent** from the fovea but have a maximum density of approximately **160000/mm²** in the perifoveal region, decreasing gradually to **3000/mm²** at the retinal periphery. There are approximately 6.3-6.8 million cones in the retina.

* Photoreceptors have a ratio with ganglion cells of **100 :1.**

* The macula lutea is a yellowish oval area **4.5 mm** (three disc diameters) long lying approximately **3 mm** lateral to the optic disc. The central area of the macula is depressed and is known as the fovea centralis; it measures **1.5 mm** in diameter. The cone density is maximal at this point (approximately **150000/m²**)

* The medial rectus has the **shortest** tendon (**3.7 mm**); that of the lateral rectus is the **longest at 8.8 mm.**

* The superior oblique pulls forward at an angle of approximately **55°** to the nasal side of the globe's visual axis with the eye in the primary position; the inferior oblique pulls at an angle of approximately **50°.**

* The profile of antibody response to HIV infection will vary between the AIDS related complex (ARC) and "fully blown" AIDS. Antibodies against envelope glycoproteins such as **gp 41, gp 120, and gp 160** are present in both the AIDS related complex and AIDS. Transition from the complex to AIDS is signalled by a decrease in antibody to core proteins such as p24, and a decrease in the T4/T8 ratio.

* Timolol is a relatively selective β1 antagonist, despite the fact that most receptors in the eye are β2 receptors. This problems is overcome by the aqueous concentrations of timolol, which are **1000 times** those required for β2 stimulation.

* A patient is said to be a "high" steroid responder if, after a **4 weeks** course of dexamethasone, their intraocular pressure is **<30 mmHg** (pretreatment pressure **< 20 mmHg).** In the general population 6% of people fall into this category but 90% of patients with open angle glaucoma are "high" responders. Non proliferative diabetic retinopathy and high myopia also shows an increased incidence of "high responders".

* The maximum volume of the conjunctival sac is **20 µl** but the normal tear volume is approximately **6-7 ml** because of the effect of blinking. This explains why only 20% of an average drop of medication (approximately **50 ml**) is retained in the conjunctival sac, the rest being lost to overflow. A tear turnover rate of **18% per minute** compounds poor retention of medication, which means that after 5 minutes only **40%** of the medication is present in the conjunctival sac. A normal Schirmer's test would produce 15-25 mm of "wetting" over a period of 5 minutes.

* Albumin accounts for 60% of tear protein. The ratio of IgG to IgA in serum is **7 :1** —this ratio is 1 : 1 in the tear film.

* The blink lasts **0.3-0.4 seconds** and occurs about **15 times** each minute.

* The anterior corneal surface has a refractive power of **48.8 diopters** and the posterior surface — **5.8 diopters : 43 diopters** in total. This accounts for 70% of the eye's refractive power.

* Both Bowman's and Descemet's membranes (adjacent to Bowman's membrane) are **10 mm** thick. Descemet's membrane is able to regenerate.

* Corneal stroma consists of water (**80%**), glycosaminoglycans (such as keratin and chondroitin sulphate), and mucopolysaccharides bind collagen and account for **5%** of the dry weight. The stroma has a very low cell count per unit volume, which explains why corneal oxygen consumption is **eight times** lower than that of the epithelium and **12 times** lower than that of the endothelium, both of which are rich in glycolytic and Krebs' cycle enzymes.

* Intraocular pressure, if **above 50 mmHg,** will cause corneal oedema.

* The optimal temporal frequency for perceiving flicker is **10 Hz.**

* Arterioles are responsible for **50%** of the peripheral vascular resistance. Capillaries have a surface area of approximately 300 m^2 but most (65%) of the blood volume is found in the veins and venules.

* The **Ferry-Porter Law** states that critical frequency varies with log mean luminance, and is true over large ranges of photopic illumination. **De Lange's name** is given to the temporal contrast sensitivity function which can be determined in a manner analogous to the spatial contrast sensitivity. For white light minimum contrast is required for a **10 Hz** flicker.

* The ratio of noradrenaline to adrenaline in the medulla is **1:6.**

* Healthy tear film has a **break-up-time** of approx **10-30 seconds.**

* The **earliest** embryonic stage at which ocular structures can be differentiated from the rest of the fetus is the embryonic plate stage (**2 weeks** stage).

* Medullation of optic nerve is completed by age **3 months.**

* At **3-4 months** of age the macula becomes slightly concave and the foveal light reflection appears.

* Most of the binocular reflexes should be well developed by **6 months** of age.

* The secretion of tears does not begin before **3-4 weeks** after birth.

* Failure of tear production by **3 months** of age demands attention.

* Stereoactivity can be shown to develop in most infants beginning at **3 months** of age.

* Failure of the nasolacrimal ducts to function by **6 months** of age needs attention.

* The corneal epithelium replaces itself about **once a week.**

* The endothelial cell density of cornea at birth is approximately **3000 cells per mm^2** and generally decreases with age.

* The cones are far fewer in number than the rods (cones —**6 million;** rods —**125 million**).

* The optic nerve consists of **1 million** axons arising from the ganglion cells of the retina.

* Descemet's membrane thickness increases with age (at birth **3 to 4.^{00}** where as in adulthood **10 to 12.^{00}**).

* The maximum intraocular pressure being found **around 6 a.m.**

* The lids remain united with each other until **7th month** of intrauterine life.

* The lens derives its nourishment upto **8th month** of foetal life by hyaloid artery; afterwards from aqueous humour.

* Visible spectrum extends form **723 m.^{00}** (Red) to **397 mμ** (Violet).

* The media of the eye are uniformity permeable to the visible rays between **600 mm* and 390 mm.**

* Cornea absorbs rays shorter than **295 m.$^{00^{\mathsf{T}}}$**

* Lens absorbs rays shorter than **350 m.^{00}.**

* Vitreous has an absorption band—maximum at **270 m.^{00}.**

* Normal eyes may differ **1-2 mm** in length.

* Corneal curvature vary from **7-8 mm.**

* The image magnification in an aphakic eye is about **30%.**

* In children younger than **2 years,** visual function is best tested by visual-evoked potential.

* Myopia of more than **6 dioptres** should be under corrected where as myopia of less than 6 dioptres should be fully corrected.

* In an aphasic eye the anterior focal length is **23 mm** whereas the posterior focal distance is **31 mm.**

* Cornea absorbs rays shorter than **295 m.ᐟ⁰⁰** whereas lens absorbs rays shorter than **350 mm.**

* The anterior focal length of the eye is **15 mm** whereas the posterior focal length of the eye is **24 mm.**

* In strong accommodation the radius of curvature of anterior surface becomes **6 mm** whereas the same with accommodation at rest is **10 mm.**

* An aphakic eye will see an increase in image size of **30%.**

* **Anterior chamber (AC) :** 1st appears at **20 mm (7 weeks)** IUL (Intrauterine length).

* The strength of the lens & its distance from the lens with a lens of **+ 13D,** the fundus of an emmetropic eye is magnified about **5 times.**

* **Optic Disc :** is Pale pink **1.5 mm** in diameter. Nearly circular (oval in astigmatism), sharp edges.

* The distance direct ophthalmoscopy is performed at a convenient distance of **22 cm.**

* In indirect ophthalmoscopy the magnification of the image of the fundus is mostly with **+ 13D lens.**

* Mydriatic effect of atropine persists for **7 days.**

* The topical nonsteroidal anti-inflammatory agent useful in allergic conjunctivitis is **Sodium cromoglycate (drops 2%, ointments 4%).**

* Pupil is tested in Horner's syndrome by i) **Adrenaline (0.1%) test ;** ii) **Cocaine (4%) test ;** iii) **Hydroxyamphetamine (1%) test.**

* Conjunctival inflammation in the newborn cannot produce a follicular reaction (because of adenoid superficial layer is devoid of lymphoid tissue until **2-3 months** postnatally).

* **Microcornea**—Cornea with diameter less than **11 mm,** a developmental defect, produces myopia, occurs in rubella syndrome, no corneal opacification, treatment not necessary except correction of refractive error.

* The average corneal endothelial cells count is **2800 cells per sq. mm** in the adult.

* A marginal ulcer, unilateral in **60-80%** of cases characterised by painful, progressive excavation of the limbus and peripheral cornea often with loss of eye in old age is called **Mooren's ulcer (Rodent ulcer, chronic serpiginous ulcer).**

* Anisocoria is a different in pupillary size and it is most commonly accepted at **0.4 mm.**

* The optimum time for vitrectomy in a patient of endophthalmitis is **24 hours** after the intravitreal injection of the culture is positive.

* The best available treatment of SRNV in age related macular degeneration when it is **200 µ** away from the foveal avascular zone is Argon green laser. Where as subretinal membranes which are located closer than **200 µ** from the foveal avascular zone are best treated by Krypton red laser.

* The best instruments for optic nerve evaluation and determination of cup/disc ratio are the direct ophthalmoscope or the **90D** volk lens.

* About 2/3rd of cases of buphthalmos can be diagnosed by the age of **6 months.**

* In children, the corneal diameter should not exceed **11 mm.** Corneal enlargement of **12 mm or greater** is strongly indicative of congenital glaucoma.

* Pilocarpine starts acting **1 hour** after instillation.

* A variation in the diurnal rhythm of IOP is significant if it is > **5.0 mm** of Hg.

* Resuscitation time of the human retina following retinal ischaemia is **1.5 hours.**

* 3 diopters of papilledema is equal to approximately **1 mm** of swelling.

* The swelling of the disc in papillitis rarely exceeds **2-3 D.**

* Two ocular conditions protect the eye from papilledema—these are high myopia (**5 to 10 diopters**) **& optic atrophy** if they are present there will be no papilledema.

* The centre of rotation of the eyes which lies in the horizontal plane is **12 mm** behind the cornia.

* The covering power may be taken to be definitely insufficiency if it falls below **20 degrees.**

* The normal field of fixation is about **50°** downwards and **45°** in all other directions.

* **5 mm** medial rectus recession in unilateral esotropia will correct about **12°squint.**

* In an emmetropic eye the angle gamma is positive which is **5°.**

* The diplopia charting is carried out at a distance of atleast **4 feet.**

* In a child with concomitant squint the surgical treatment is usually undertaken **4-5 years** of age.

* The ideal age at which to begin therapy of strabismus is **6 months.**

* Sympathetic ophthalmia occurs **4-6 weeks** after injury.

* A magnetic foreign body in the vitreous of retina is removed with an electromagnet by posterior route **5 mm** behind the limbus.

* Needling of the after cataract is advised for the presence of after cataract blocking the pupillary area following extracapsular extraction of lens (This operation is performed **5-6 weeks** after cataract operation when the eye becomes quiet).

* No facial and ciliary blocks are necessary for Discission operation (for children below **5 years,** general anaesthesia is preferable).

* The corneoscleral stitches are removed in cataract extraction after **4 weeks.**

* An artificial eye of plastic should be worn after **2 weeks** of surgery.

* An artificial eye of glass or plastic should not be worn less than **2 weeks after excision.**

* Late failure of penetrating keratoplasty is most frequently due to **Allograft reaction. (about 50% cases occur within first 6 months postoperatively).**

* If diagnosis of Amaurosis fugax due to transient retinal ischaemia is missed, **40% to 50%** of all untreated cases will develop blindness or severe visual loss.
* The prevalence of blindness in India is estimated at **1.5%** for the whole country.
* Active conjunctival xerosis and Bitot's spot begin to resolve within **2-5 days,** and mostly will disappear by **2 weeks.**
* Average age of diagnosis of retinoblastoma is **18 month** **after 7 years of age).**
* Levator muscle in an adult can raise the lid by approx **15 mm.**
* Ratio of photoreceptors with ganglion cell is **100 :1**
* Ciliary process are formed at **3 months.**
* Ora serrata is fully developed at **6 months** of gestational age.
* Optic vesicle is usually forms by day 25 of gestation
* Upper tarsal plate centrally is **2 times** thick than that of lower one.
* Maximum density of rods in perifoveal region is **1,60,000** mm^2
* Average diurral variation in IOP in glaucomatous eye is approx **10 mm.**
* Flickering sensation to be cone driven must be more than **30 Hz**
* Gene for short (blue) wavelength is found in chromosome 7.
* Number of classes of colour defectives is **8.**
* Pupilary dilatation in dark adaptation can account for an increase in sensitivity of **1.3 log unit.**
* Accommodation is absent by the age of atleast 60 years.
* Vitreous does not transmit the light below **300 nm.**
* Optimal temporal frequency for perceiving flicker is **10 Hz.**
* Retina contains approx **120 million** rodes.
* Stereopsis is poor beyond **20 °** from fovea.
* If the inferior rectus is hooked in attempt to recess it 5 mm, the new insertion of limbus into sclera will be 11mm.
* Conjunctiva fuses with Tenon's capsule **3 mm** from the limbus.
* Lower punctum lies **6.5 mm** from the medial canthus and the superior punctum slightly medial at **6mm** from medial canthus.

* Vertical diameter of eyeball is **23 mm**, horizontal diameter is **23.5 mm** and A.P. diameter is **24 mm.**

* Corneal epithelium is 50-60 μm thick and is 10% of the corneal thickness.

* **Bowman's membrane** is 10 mm thick, containing a matrix of collagen fibrils.

* Descement's membrane is 6-10 mm thick.

* Sclera is made-up of approx **68%** water and remains opaque with values between 40% and 80%.

* Pars plicata is made up of 70-80 folds forming the ciliary processes.

* The lens fibres are **12 mm long,** 13 shaped fibres tightly packed and, attached to end others, by interdigiting ball and socket and tongue and groove joints in the cortex and nucleus respectively.

* Retina contains approx **6.5 million** cones 1 lac of which are present in the fovea and 120 million rods.

* In striate cortex, **IV layer** is the thickest.

* Accommodation is well developed by the age of **2 months.**

* Turnover time of water in vitreous is **10-15 min.**

* Predominant collagen in vitreous is **type II.**

* **Arden ratio** (between the light peak and dark trough) in EOG in normal person is usually greater than at least **180%.**

* Vitreous weighs about **3.9 gm.**

* Staph. epidermidis is the **most common** organism isolated from intraocular contents of eye with postoperative endophthalmitis.

* Accommodative power of a 2 year old is approx **20 diopters.**

* The lateral rectus has the **longest** tendon length (**8.8 mm**) followed by the superior rectus (**5.8 mm**), then the inferior rectus (**5.5 mm**) and lastly the medial rectus (**3.7 mm**).

* The medial rectus inserts into the sclera closest to the limbus (**5.5 mm**), followed by the inferior rectus (**6.5 mm**), then lateral rectus (**6.9 mm**) and last, the superior rectus (**7.7 mm**).

* Superior obliques has a muscle length of approx 32mm.

* The central retinal vein leaves the optic nerve **10 mm** from the eyeball.

* **75 percent** of myaesthenic present with ocular involvement (diplopia or ptosis).

* Vitreous osmolality is **280-322 mOsm/kg** .

* Vitreous to plasma ascorbic acid is **9 : 1.**

* Rhodopsin has a half life of **420 years.**

* In retina, although 60% of glucose is metabolised anaerobically and only 25% is metabolised aerobically (contributing 90% of energy production).

* The fibres in lens are closely packed with a distance of **100/200A°**

* Anaerobic glycolysis produces **60%** of lens energy and aerobic glycolysis **40%** of lens energy (yielding 36 ATP per glucose molecule) 15% of glucose is metabolised via HMP shunt, 80% of lens glucose is metabolised by anaerobic glycolysis and 4% by aerobic glycolysis.

* Vitreous transmits upto **90%** of visible light between **300 and 400 nm**. It does not transmit light below 300 nm.

* Corneal epithelial turnover is within **7 days** (once a week).

* Collagen forms 71% of dry weight of corneal stroma and is mainly type I. There are however lesser amounts of type III to type VI collagen also present.

* Corneal endothelial cell density at birth is approx **3500-4000 cells/mm^2**. The adult cornea has a cell density between 1400 and 2500 cells/mm^2. Corneal transplants may have less than 1000 cells/mm^2 and still remain clear with normal functions. The **critical level** for adequate corneal function is between 400 and 700 cells/mm^2 approx.

* Corneal endothelium pumps fluid into the anterior chamber at a rate of **10μl/h.** This amounts to approx **8%** of the aqueous production rate.

* Insulin levels in aqueous are 3% of those in plasma and increase by a factor of 10 postprandially.

* Aqueous production and IOP have a diurnal variation with a peak between 7 and 9 AM.

* Concentration of glucose in aqueous is 80% of that in plasma.

* Pupil diameter can range from 1 to 9 mm.

* Horner's after the age of 2 years usually does not cause heterochromia. Hydroxyamphetamine test has a diagnostic accuracy of 84% for post- ganglionic lesions and 97% for central or preganglionic lesions. In it, hydroxyamphetamine produces mydriasis in central and preganglionic . Horner's but fails to dilate the eye in postganglionic Horner's syndrome.

* Protein binding of fluorescein in blood is **70-85%**.

* Probing of nasolacrimal duct should not be done till the age of **6 months** and preferably for **12 months.**

* Cilia are normally replaced every **3-5 months** and are replaced in **two months** of forcibly removed.

* Bell's phenomenon is absent in **10%** of the population.

* Corneal blink reflex consists of an ipsilateral disynaptic fast phase with a latency of **10-15 ms** and a second slower bilateral multisynaptic phase of **20-35 ms** latency.

* At photopic levels, blinking of upto **3 ms** duration shows no discontinuity of visual perception.

* Corneal stroma consists of **78%** water or **3.45 parts** weight of water to one part solid .

* Cornea transmits radiation at 310 nm (in UV) to 2500 nm (infrared). It is most sensitive at **270 nm** which can result in photokeratitis.

* Macula fully develops by **4-6 months** of age.

* Sclera is about **1 mm** thick at its thickest portion.

* Normal diameter of cornea is about **13 mm.**

* **4 images** formed by four reflecting surfaces of eye (ant. and post. part of cornea and lens) when strongly illuminated source falls on the eye, are called Purkinje-Sanson images.

* Retinoblastoma is commonest in 0 to 5 years (common in both sexes) and usually unilateral. Rossettes (True and Pseudo) are seen.

* Superior and inferior recti makes an angle of 23° in AP diameter and superior and inferior oblique makes 51°.

* Size of different recti are — SLIM (8 mm, 7 mm, 6.5 mm 5.5. mm for different recti as indicated in Mnemonic).
* The dioptric power of cornea in adults is **43 D.**
* The thickness of lens in an adult is **4.25 mm.**
* The length of eyeball in an adult is **23 to 24 mm.**
* The normal refractive power of an emmetropic eye is **58 dioptre.**
* Sclera is perforated by **4 Vertex veins.**
* Aquous humour (volume is **0.25 cc** in ant. chamber and **0.06 c.c.** in posterior) has more Na+ and vitamin-C as compared to plasma but has negligible protein.
* Normal IOP is **16-23 mm Hg.**
* Thickness of retina is **0.5 mm** near optic disc, **0.2 mm** at equator and **0.1 mm** most anteriorly.
* The size of optic disc is **1.5 mm.**
* Extent of field of vision is 60° nasally as well as above, **75°** below and **100°** on temporal side.
* Macula is situated **2-2.5 disc dimeters** on the temporal side of optic disc and **1 disc diameter** is **1.5 mm** on an average.
* Each individual letter on Snellen's test subtend an angle of **5 minutes** whereas each component part of letter subtends an angle of **1 minute.**
* A difference of refraction of **4 diopters** between eyes cause an image size difference of more than **7%**, results in diplopia.
* Spontaneous regression of a strawberry haemangioma may occur up to **5 years** of age.

OCULAR DIMENSIONS AND BASIC OPTICAL DATA
(Adult eyes : Average figures from multiple surveys)

Globe
* circumference : 75 mm
* diameter : 24 mm
* volume : 6.5 cc
* weight : 7.5 g

Cornea
* diameter (external)
  -horizontal : 11.75 mm
  -vertical : 10.55 mm

Iris (Most parameters variable)
* pupillary sphincter
    -width 0.75-0.8 mm
* pupillary diameter
    -range 1.1-8.0 mm (actual)
    1.3-9.0 mm (apparent)
    -average : 3.5 mm (actual)
    4.0 mm (apparent)
* radius of curvature (central)
    -anterior 7.8 mm
    -posterior 6.5 mm
* thickness (full)
    -central 0.58 mm
    -peripheral : 1.33
* weight : 1.80 mg
* refractive index : 1.33
    -thickness
    -epithelium : 50-100 μ
    -Bowman's : 10-13 μ
    (central to peripheral)
    -stroma 0.6-0.9 mm
    (central to peripheral)
    -Descemet's 5-10 μ
    -endothelium : 5-6 μ (height)
    20 μ (width)
    1600-4000 cells/mm^2 (density)

Sclera
* thickness
    -limbus 0.83 mm
    -sub tendon : 0.30 mm
    -equator : 5.50 mm
    -posterior pole : 1.00-1.35 mm

Ciliary Body

* width (total)
  — nasal and superior : 4.5-5.2 mm
  — temporal and inferior : 5.6-6.3 mm
* pars plicata (corona ciliaris)
  — width : 2.0 mm
* pars plana (orbicularis ciliaris)
  — width : 3.6-4.0 mm
* ciliary processes
  — number 70-80
  — width : 0.5 mm
  — length : 2.0 mm
  — height : 0.8-1.0 mm

Lens

* equatorial diameter : 9.0 mm
* sagittal diameter : 4.0-4.14 mm (increases with age)
* weight
  -20-30 yrs old : 0.174 g
  -80-90 yrs old : 0.266 g
* radius of curvature
  -anterior 8.4-1.8 mm (average 10.0)
  -posterior : 4.6-7.5 mm (average 6.0)

Anterior Chamber

* depth : 3.6 mm
* volume : 0.25 cc (approx.)

Choroid

* thickness
  -posterior pole :
  0.10-0.30 mm
    -equator : 0.50 mm
    -ora serrata : 0.06 mm

Optic Nerve

* number of fibers : 1 million (estimate)

* length
  — globe to chiasm : 35-55 mm
  — intraocular : 1.0 mm
  — oribital : 25 mm
  — canalicular : 4-10 mm
  — intracranial : 10 mm
* diameter
  — intraocular : 1.6 mm
  — intraorbital : 3.0-4.0 mm
  — intracranial : 4.0-7.0 mm

Optic Chiasma

* dimensions
  — sagittal : 8.0 mm
  — transverse : 12.0 mm
  — dorso-ventral : 4.0-7.0 mm

Vitreous

* volume approximately 5 cc

Retina

* thickness
  — at disc : 0.56 mm
  — equator : 0.18 mm
  — ora serrata : 0.10 mm
* distance retinal periphery-limbus
  — nasal : 5.0 mm
  — temporal : 6.5 mm
* number of rods : 120 million (estimate)
* number of cones : 7 million (estimate)
* vascular
  — diameter of veins at disc : 125 μ
  — diameter cap. free zone 500 μ

Sella Turcica

* A-P diameter : 5-16 mm
* vertical depth : 4-12 mm
* volume : 250-1100 mm^3
  mean —600 mm^3

* angle of muscle (tendon) with A-P axis of globe
  — S.R. : 23°
  — I.R. : 23°
  — S.O : 54°
  — I.O : 51°
* trochlea : 6.0 mm x 4.0 mm

Orbit

* volume : 29.0-30.0 cc
* height at entrance : 35.0 mm
* width at entrance : 40.0 mm
* extraorbital width (lateral margin-lateral margin) : 100.0 mm
* angle of lateral/medial wall : 45°
* angle of lateral/lateral wall : 90°
  Optic canal
  — length : 4.0-9.0 mm
  — width : 4.0-6.0 mm

Eye Lids

* tarsus (upper)
  — height (centrally) : 10.0-12.0 mm
  — length (at margin) : 29.0 mm
  — thickness : 1.0 mm
* tarsus (lower)
  — height (centrally) : 5.0 mm
  — length and thickness as for upper
* palpebral fissure
  — length : 30.0 mm
  — height : 15 mm
* Meibomian glands (tarsal glands)
  — number (upper lid) : 30-40
* Krause glands
  — number (upper lid) : 20
  — number (lower lid) : 8
* Wolfring glands
  — at superior border of upper tarsus

* **Blinking**
  — each blink lasts : 0.3 sec.
  — average rate : 12/min

Lacrimal excretory system

* puncta
  — diameter : 0.2-0.3 mm
* canaliculi
  — vertical length : 1.5 mm
  — horizontal length : 8.5 mm
  — total length : 10.0 mm
* lacrimal sac
  — width : 4.8 mm
  — height ; 10.0-12.0 mm
  — fundus (above medial canthal tendon) : 3.0-5.0 mm
* nasolacrimal duct
  — length : intraosseus : 12.4 mm
     intrameatal : 5.3 mm

Tears

* pH : 7.4
* secretion /24 hrs : 1.0 g (1.2 μL/min)
* Schirmer test (What man No. 41 filter paper 5 X30 mm); 10-25 mm/ 5 min.
* osmotic pressure : equiv. to 0.9-0.95% NaCl.
* tear film layers
  — superficial oily : Meibomian and Zeis glands.
  — middle watery: lacrimal and accessory lacrimal glands.
  — deep mucoid: goblet cells and crypts of Henle.
* **Composition**
  — 98-99% water
  — K+ several times than serum
  — Proteins : 0.2-0.6% (higher in emotions)
  — Refractive index : 1. 33
  — Isotonic (closed eye)
  — hypertonic (open eye)
  — Serous component absent in first 4 weeks of life.
     Normal levels in 6 months.

COMMONEST IN OPHTHALMOLOGY

* The **most common** cause of blindness is cataract
* The **most common** cause of blindness in adults is cataract.
* The **most common** cause of blindness in children is Vitamin A deficiency.
* The **most common** cause of ocular morbidity is Refractive error.
* The **most common** cause of Low vision is Refractive error.
* **Most common** site of metastasis for intraocular malignant melanoma is—Liver.
* **Most common** type of keratitis—Herpes simplex keratitis.
* **Most common** cause of subluxation of lens—Trauma.
* **Most common** form of uveitis—Idiopathic.
* **Most common** cause of acute retinal necrosis syndrome is — Herpes infection in AIDS.
* **Most common** cause of viral corneal ulcer—H. simplex
* **Most common** cause of viral conjunctivitis—Adeno virus.
* **Most common** cause of bilateral papilloedema—Brain tumor.
* **Most common** site for concussion cataract—Posterior cortex.
* **Most common** bacteria causing central corneal ulcer—Pneumococci.
* **Most common** site for lodgement of intraocular foreign body—vitreous.
* **Most common** manifestation of maternal rubella—Cataract.
* **Most common** intraocular cyst is —Traumatic.
* The **most common** lesion of choroid as a result of myopia or obliterative vasosclerosis is **Central Choroidal Atrophy.**

* The **most common** form of cataract is the **commonest** congenital cataract causing visual impairment (otherwise blue dot cataract is the **commonest** congenital type).

* Most common postoperative complication of extracapsular cataract extraction is posterior capsule thickening.

* The most commonly encountered developmental cataract is anterior axial embryonal cataract.

* The **most common** form of glaucoma is primary open angle glaucoma.

* The **most common** associated congenital anomalies with Buphthalmos is Neurofibromatosis.

* The **most common** complication following trephining operation for glaucoma is secondary infection.

* The **commonest** hazard following surgery of congestive glaucoma is malignant glaucoma.

* The **commonest** side-effect of acetazolamide is numbness and tingling of fingers and toes.

* **Most common** site in eye for secondary metastasis —Choroid.

* **Most specific** ophthalmic diagnostic procedure in Sjogren's syndrome is —Slit lamp examination of cornea after Rose Bengal staining.

* **Most common** manifestation of Behcet's syndrome is recurrent aphthous ulceration.

* **Most dreaded** complication of Behcet's syndrome is — Hypopyon uveitis.

* **Most common** lid swelling—Chalazion, Meibomian cyst.

* **Most common** malignant tumor of eye lid—Basal cell carcinoma (Rodent ulcer).

* **Most common** malignant intraocular tumor in adult is—Malignant melanoma.

* Cavernous haemangioma is the **most common benign orbital tumour,** growth rate may be accelerated by pregnancy, may give rise to visual loss without much proptosis, high internal reflectivity is seen on ultrasonography.

* Rhabdomyosarcoma is the **most common primary malignant orbital tumour** in children.

* Astigmatism is without a doubt the **most common** refractive error corrected today.

* **Most common** cause of myopia is axial myopia (due to too long length of the eye ball).

* **Most common** cause of hypermetropia is axial hypermetropia (due to abnormal shortness of antero-posterior diameter of globe).

* The **commonest** symptom complained of by an aphakic wearing aphakic correction is **pincushion distortion.**

* The **commonest age** of presentation of myopia is between 5-10 years.

* The **commonest** type of astigmatism encountered in general population is astigmatism against the rule.

* The most commonly used tests for colour vision testing are the polychromatic plates of **Ishihara, Stilling, or Hardy-Rand-Ritler.**

* The device most commonly used by the general physician for measuring IOP is **Schiotz tonometer.**

* The most commonly used ophthalmoscopy is being hand-held ophthalmoscope designed for direct magnified (14 X) view.

* The **commonest** eye disorders in childhood are **squint and obstruction of the nasolacrimal duct.**

* The most common indentation tonometer in clinical use is that of **Schiotz.**

* Conjunctivitis is the **most common** eye disease in the western hemisphere.

* The **commonest** bacteria responsible for an acute mucopurulent conjunctivitis is **Staphylococcus aureus.**

* The **most common** cause of ophthalmia neonatorum is **Chlamydia trachomatis.**

* The **most common** site of corneal ulceration in ophthalmia neonatorum is **below the centre of the cornea.**

* The commonest causes of acute catarrhal conjunctivitis are the **Pneumococcus** (in temperate climates) & **H. aegypticus** (in warm climates).

* The **most common** cause of red eye is **acute conjunctivitis.**

* The **most common** cause (now) of phlyctenulosis is **Staphylococci.**

* The **commonest cyst** of conjunctiva is **Lymphatic cyst.**

* The **most common** cause of phlyctenulosis is a hypersensitive response to microbial proteins (staphylococci).

* The **commonest** micro-organism responsible for a neonatal conjunctivitis is TRIC agents.

* In trachoma corneal ulcer occur anywhere but are **commonest** at the **advancing edge of the pannus.**

* The **most common** cause of corneal edema is increased intraocular pressure.

* The commonest cause of failure in treatment of hypopyon ulcer is the development of secondary glaucoma (a complication which usually occurs in elderly people).

* The **commonest** corneal dystrophy is **Reis-Buckler's type.**

* Epithelial basement membrane dystrophies are seen most commonly after the age of 30.

* Keratoconus most commonly progresses slowly over a number of decades.

* The **most common** cranial nerve palsy affected by herpes zoster ophthalmicus is third cranial nerve.

* Rheumatoid arthritis is the most common collagen vascular disorder to affect the peripheral cornea.

* The **most common** ocular complication of SLE is punctate epithelial keratopathy.

* **Commonest** cause of corneal opacity is healed corneal ulcer.

* Microcystic dystrophy (**Cogan's mapdot-finger print** or epithelial basement membrane) is the **most common** dystrophy of cornea seen in clinical practice (macular dystrophy is least common).

* Disciform keratitis is the **commonest** complication of HSV infection.

* Tuberculosis is the **commonest** cause of uveitis.

* Synchysis (liquefaction) and syneresis (collapse) are the two **most common** degenerative changes in the vitreous gel.

* Posterior staphyloma is **most commonly** seen in pathological myopia.

* The **commonest** complication in recurrent uveitis is Glaucoma.

* The **most common** complication of pars planitis is complicated cataract.

* The **commonest** cause of iridoschisis is senile atrophy.

* Haemangioma of choroid is **most commonly** associated with Sturge-Weber's syndrome.

* The **most commonly** encountered hazard after long term pilocarpine instillation is visual blur.

* Diabetes is the **most common** cause of cotton wool spots.

* Retinal haemorrhage is the change **most commonly** associated with hypertension.

* The **most common** cause of traction retinal detachment are proliferative retinopathies (diabetic retinopathy) or penetrating injuries.

* Autosomal recessive is the **most common** mode of inheritance of retinitis pigmentosa.

* Embolization is the **most common** cause of obstruction to the retinal circulation.

* Retinal branch artery occlusion is most commonly caused by emboli.

* Pseudoxanthoma elasticum is the most common systemic disorder associated with angioid streaks.

* The **most common** syndrome associated with retinitis pigmentosa is Laurence-Moon-Biedl syndrome.

* The **commonest** cause of spontaneous vitreous haemorrhage is proliferative diabetic retinopathy.

* Most common inheritance of pigmentary retinal dystrophy is recessive.

* The most common quadrant to have retinal holes is superotemporal.
* Retinal detachment is common in aphakia and myopia.
* The **commonest** variety of primary pigmentary retinal dystrophy is without any family history.
* Retinoschisis most commonly occurs in lower temporal quadrants.
* Homonymous hemianopia is the **commonest** form of field loss & may be due to a lesion anywhere between the occipital lobe & the chiasma.
* Accident or factitious instillation of drug that cause pupillary dilation is seen **most commonly** in persons in medical settings.
* The chromophobe adenoma is the **most common** primary intracranial tumor producing neuro-ophthalmological features.
* The **most common** ocular manifestations of multiple sclerosis are the result of demyelination of the optic nerve and brainstem.
* The **most common** conditions that affect the III CN are aneurysm, tumor, inflammation and vascular disease.
* The **most common** condition to affect the IV CN is **trauma** (second most common cause is diabetes).
* By far the **most common** cause of anterior ischaemic optic neuropathy is giant cell artheritis.
* Internuclear ophthalmoplegia (INO) is most commonly associated with multiple sclerosis.
* The two **most common** ocular signs of myasthenia gravis are drooping eyelid (ptosis) and extrocular muscle weakness (causing strabismus).
* Vision loss is the **most common** facial symptom of optic nerve glioma.
* **Most commonly** suppression occurs in strabismus patient, (where abnormal alignment of the eye causes different areas of the two retinas to be stimulated; a condition that would result in double vision or diplopia.
* The **commonest** cause of binocular diplopia is paralysis of extraocular muscles.

* The **most common** cause of paretic strabismus is due to haemorrhagic thrombotic lesion in the midbrain associated with arteriosclerosis or diabetes.

* In pressure paralysis the nerve most commonly involved is Abducens (6th) cranial nerve.

* The **common** cause of bilateral internuclear ophthalmoplegia is multiple sclerosis

* The **most common** type of strabismus is **Esotropia (manifest convergent strabismus).**

* The **most common** and most virulent fungal disease (phycomycosis) involving the orbit are caused by organisms of the class **Phycomycetes.**

* The most common fungal genera causing phycomycosis are mucor (mucormycosis) and Rhizopus.

* Marginal blepharitis is the **most common** disorder of the lids.

* Surgery is by far the **most common** method of treatment for chalazion.

* Congenital ptosis is the **commonest** form of ptosis affiction.

* Meibomian cyst (Chalazion) is the **most common** lid swelling.

* The **most common** cause of congenital ptosis is defective development of levator palpebrae superioris.

* The **commonest** malignant growth of the lid is basal cell carcinoma.

* Chronic dacryocystitis is more common abnormality of the lacrimal passage is an obstruction at nasolacrimal duct.

* The **commonest** site of obstruction in epiphora occurring in an adult is junction of the sac and the nasolacrimal duct.

* In the orbital cellulitis, the **most common** nasal sinus from where extension of inflammation occurs is ethmoidal sinus.

* Pseudotumour of the orbits is **commonest** between the age group of 40-60 years.

* Mucocele of accessory sinus of the nose affecting the orbit most commonly occurs in Frontal sinus.

* The **most common** cause of intermittent exophthalmos is orbital vertices.

* The **most frequent** cause of pulsating exophthalmos is carotico-cavernous fistula.

* The **commonest** cause of canaliculitis is Actinomyces.

* The primary tumour of the orbit most commonly presenting with proptosis is cavernous haemangioma.

* The **commonest** primary malignant tumour of the orbit in a child is Rhabdomyosarcoma.

* The **commonest** histological type of rhabdomyosarcoma of the orbit is embryonal type.

* The **commonest** finding in anaemia is pallor of the tarsal conjunctiva.

* The eye is most commonly involved in the severe bullous form of erythema multiforme disease (in which mucous membrane is involved—the Steven-Johnson syndrome).

* The **most common** ophthalmic complaints of acoustic neuroma are diplopia & blurred vision (the **most common** non-ocular symptom is unilateral hearing loss).

* Toxoplasmosis is probably the **most common** cause of posterior chorioretinitis.

* Thyrotoxicosis is the **commonest** cause of proptosis.

* The **commonest** extraocular muscle palsy in tabes dorsalis is oculomotor nerve.

* The **commonest** lid sign of dysthyroid exophthalmos is Dalrymple's sign.

* The **commonest** ocular sign of hypothyroidism is cataract.

* The **commonest** feature of Waardenburg's syndrome is lateral displacement of both medial canthi and lacrimal puncta.

* Basal cell carcinoma is the most common human malignancy (90% occur in head & neck and of these 10% involve eye lid).

* Basal cell carcinoma is the **most common** malignant tumour of the eye lid (90% of all cases).

* The two external beams most commonly used to treat lid neoplasms are orthovoltage **photons** and megavoltage electrons.

* Squamous cell carcinoma is the **commonest** malignant lesion of the conjunctiva.

* Choroidal malignant melanoma is the **most common** primary intraocular tumor of adults.
* The **most common** adult iris lesions are naevi, melanoma and cysts.
* The **most common** initial presentation of von-Hippel-Lindau syndrome is decreased vision in the second or third decade of life.
* **Most common** benign ocular tumor of infancy is capillary hemangioma.
* Rhabdomyosarcoma is the **most common** primary orbital malignancy (accounts for 5% of all childhood malignancies).
* Most common presentations of orbital rhabdomyosarcoma is ptosis or lid mass.
* Most commonly, children who develop either orbital osteogenic sarcomas or leiomyosarcomas had bilateral retinoblastoma approximately 10 years previously.
* The **commonest** orbital ocular vascular tumor presenting in children is lymphangioma.
* Cavernous haemangioma is the **most common** adult intracranial (the volume surrounded by the extraocular muscles) tumor.
* Optic nerve sheath meningioma is the most common adult optic nerve tumor.
* The second most common sinus process that involves the adult orbit is malignant squamous cell carcinoma with contiguous spread.
* Metastatic tumours of the orbit—
  * In woman—breast cancer is most common.
  * In man —lung cancer is most common.
  * In children—neuroblastoma is most common.
* Pathologically the **most common** cell type in choroidal malignant melanoma is mixed cell type.
* The **most common** mode of metastasis of retinoblastoma is by direct extension, by continuity to the optic nerve.
* The **most common** site of metastasis of retinoblastoma is brain in the intracranial cavity.

* The **commonest** histological type of rhabdomyosarcoma of the orbit is embryonal.

* The **commonest** tumour of the lacrimal gland is benign mixed tumour.

* The **most common** malignant tumor of mesenchymal origin in the orbit is **Rhabdomyosarcoma.**

* The **most common** type of injury to iris is rupture of pupillary margin.

* The **most common** site for rupture of the eyeball is **along the limbus.**

* The **most common** cause of deterioration of visual acuity in **4-12 weeks** after intracapsular cataract extraction is cystoid macular oedema.

* The common material used for manufacture of intraocular lens is PMMA.

* The **most common** complication of intraocular lens implantation is posterior capsule thickening.

* The **most common** method used for treating the retinal hole is cryotherapy.

* The **commonest** complication in exfoliation of the lens capsule is Glaucoma.

* **Commonest** complication of posterior intraocular implant is dislocation.

* The **most common** presentation of functional visual loss is constricted visual fields or decreased visual acuity in one or both eyes.

* **Most commonly** employed colour vision test to detect colour blindness is Isochromatic charts.

* Glaucoma is the second **most common** cause of vision loss in the elderly population.

* **Most common** primary malignant tumor of orbit in childhood is Rhabdomyosarcoma.

* **Most common** benign tumor of lacrymal gland is Mixed-Cell Tumor.

* **Most common** Adjacent tumor which invades the orbit is Sq. cell carcinoma of maxillary antrum.

* **Most common** type of Rhabdomysarcoma is embryonal type.

* **Most common** tumor of Lacrimal sac is transitional cell tumor.

* **Most common** part of orbit involved by Rhabdomyosarcoma is superonasal quadrant.

* **Most common** tumor of conjunctiva is naevus (benign pigment tumor).

* **Most common** epibulbar tumor in children is Choriostoma.

* **Most common** site of conjunctival dermoid is **inferotemporal part** of the Limbus.

* **Most common** site of epibulbar osseous choriostoma is **Superotemporal part** of bulbar conjunctiva.

* **Most common** site of squamous papilloma of conjunctiva in children is inferior fornix.

* **Most common** melanocytic tumor of conjunctiva is circumscribed nervus.

* **Most common** site of malignant melanoma of conjuctiva is Limbus

* **Most common** site of **local** metastasis from conjunctival malignant melanoma is regional lymph nodes.

* **Most common** site of **distant** metastasis from conjuctival malignant melanoma is Brain.

* **Most common** adjacent tumor from which conjunctiva is secondarily involved is Sebaceous Gland Carcinoma of the Eyelid.

* **Most common** caruncular tumors are papilloma & nervus.

* **Most common** site of benign Oncocytoma in eye is lacrymal glands.

* **Most common** benign tumor of eyelid is squamous papilloma.

* **Most common** malignant tumor of eyelid is basal cell carcinoma.

* **Most common** mesenchymal tumor of eyelid is Hemangioma.

* **Most common** site of sebaceous gland carcinoma (Meibomian cell carcinoma) is upper lid.

* **Most common** vascular tumor of eyelid is capillary hemangioma.

* **Most common** primary intraocular tumor is malignant melanoma of choroid in adults.

* **Most common** clinical form of retinoblastoma is Somatic-nonhereditory.

* **Most common** genetic form of retinoblastoma is somatic-nonhereditory.

* **Most common** endogenous mutagen in retinoblastoma is 5-methylcytosine.

* **Most common** cause of glaucoma in patient with retinoblastoma is Iris neovascularization.

* **Most common** cause of **pseudoretinoblastoma** is persistent hyperplastic primary vitreous.

* **Most common** hereditary cause of pseudoretinoblastoma is Noorie's disease.

* **Most common** site of metastasis in retinoblastoma is —bone (skull most commonly).

* **Most common** disease associated with retinal and optic nerve astrocytoma is Tuberous Sclerosis (Bourneville's disease, Epiloia).

* **Most common** site for retinal pigment epithelial **hamartoma** is Juxtapupillary region.

* **Most common** presentation of ocular reticulum cell sarcoma (Histiocytic Lymphoma) is **Bilateral vitreous** infiltration.

* **Most common** site for basal cell carcinoma of conjuctiva is Plica-Semilunaris.

* Beta soluble crystalline protein is the **commonest** type in lens.

* The **commonest** cause of proptosis is dysthyroid disease.

* A meibomian cyst is the **commonest** type of lid swelling.

* Diabetic retinopathy is the **commonest** in middle life.

* Chronic open angle glaucoma is the **commonest** type of glaucoma

* The **most common** cause of blindness in persons over 65 (in developed countries) is macular degeneration.

* Inflammation is the **commonest** disease of uvea.

* **Most common** type of cataract is senile type.

* Rheumatoid arthritis is the **commonest** disease associated with true defective tear production.
* Steroids react with amino groups of lens crystallines to precipitate the formation of disulphide bonds leading to protein aggregation and cataract (Post. subcapsular is **most common**).
* Commonest cause of binocular diplopia is paralysis of extra ocular muscles.
* Zonular or lamellar cataract is the **commonest** congenital cataract causing visual impairment, otherwise blue dot cataract is the commonest congenital type.
* Tuberculosis is the **commonest** cause of uveitis.
* Thyrotoxicosis is the **commonest** cause of proptosis.
* Cataract is the **commonest** cause of blindness in India.
* The **commonest** organism responsible for corneal ulcer is pneumococcus.
* Epibulbar dermoid is **commonest** congenital tumor of conjunctiva.
* Basal cell carcinoma is the **most common** malignant lid tumour.
* The most common cause for failure to reattack the retina is **open retinal break (Pre-operative or operative)**.

IMPORTANT POINTS TO BE REMEMBERED

* Mucopolysacharide hyaluronic acid is present in vitreous humor .

* Orbital varices produce intermittent proptosis and diplopia during periods of venous hypertension such as coughing, straining or leaning forward.

* Lamina cribrosa is absent in **morning glory syndrome** (name after flower) associated with coloboma of optic disc. In this disc falls within excavation. In affects girls proferably and is mostly unilateral.

* Transport of ascorbic acid in lens is done by myoinositol.

* Chronic papilloedema is asssociated with decreased axonal flow, ECF increased and destruction of axon.

* Free radicals in lens are handled by Vit C, Vit E and catalase. SOD, glutathione peroxidase and catalase are enzymes involved.

* **Best disease** in autosomal dominant

* Hyaluronic acid in seen in vitreous, synovium and loose connective tissue. Dermatan sulfate is widest.

* In distribution Karatan sulfate-I is in cornea and keratan sulfate II is in connective tissue.

* Superior oblique is last muscle to be rendered akinetic in retrobulbar anaesthetic block as IV cranial nerve is outside the muscle cone.

* For iris neovascularization, panretinal photo coagulation is used.

* The most important factor in the prevention of endophthalmitis in cataract surgery is preoperative preparation with povidine iodine.

* A recurrent chalazion should be subjected to histopathologic evaluation to exclude the possibility of sebaceous cell carcinoma.

* The crystalline lens derive its nourishment from aquous and humor by chemical exchanges.

* Band shaped keratopathy is caused by calcium and is seenin hypercalcemia, chronic uteitis in adults, Still's disease, pthisis bulbi, chronic keratitis or glaucoma, ocular trauma.

* Mucin layer tear film deficiency occurs in herpetic keratitis.

* Prognostic factors in choroidal melanoma are size, small is better location (in irris has best outcome), age (younger than 60 beter outcome) extra ocular extension (poor), cytolosy (epitheloid) type has worst prognosis).

* Non herigable (somatic) retinoblastoma accounts for 60% of cases.

* Dangerous area of eyeball is ciliary body.

* Ionic pump in corneal endothelium maintains hydration by cellular metabolism. It can be blocked by inhibition of anaerobic glycolysis.

* WHO defines low vision children as visual acquity 6/18 or 6/60 in better eye with best correction.

* The major function of major intrinsic protein 26 (MIP-26) is transport of water in lens.

* Final common pathway for horizontal gaze involves abducent nucleus.

* Sarcoidosis is associated with band keratopathy.

* Persistent primary hyperplastic vitreous is associated with band keratopathy

* Persistent primary hyperplastic vitreous is associated with Patau syndrome.

Salient points about Morning glory syndrome :

* Morning glory syndrome is associated with colobom of optic disc with central excavation .it occurs due to anomalous tunnel shaped expansion of distal portion of optic stalk.

* Morning glory syndrome (named after the flower) is a rare congenital anomaly of the optic papilla (region where the optic nerve emerges in the eye).

* It affects girls preferentially and is mostly unilateral. The diagnosis may be established on presentation of a strabismus, an amblyopia (impaired vision), a nystagmus, or a leucocoria (white pupil).

* Refraction anomalies are not uncommon: myopia, astigmatism, hypermetropia.

* At eye fundoscopy there is a large papilla with a tunnel-shaped optic nerve head with a white dot in the center, an elevated ring of pigment aorund the disc, and thin and straight vessels radiating out from the ring like spokes. Arteries and veins are not distinguishable. The peripheral retina and fovea are normal.

* Vision in the affected eye is severely impaired and non-evolutive.

* **Morning glory syndrome** is often associated with severe anomalies of the central nervous system (basal transphenoidal encephalocele, agensis of corpus callosum, defect of the floor of the sella turcica, chiasma agenesis). with endocrine, renal or respiratory anomalies, with one of the components of the charge association (Coloboma, Heart defects, Atresia of the choanae, Retarded growth, Ear anomalies), and in some cases with hypertelorism or cleft palate.

* There is an increased risk of retinal detachment.

* **Mutations in the PAX6 gene** have identified in families with the genetic syndromes including the Morning glory anomaly.

* There is no treatment for this anomaly, associated anomalies should be looked for in order to treat them when possible.

Cause of Mucin deficiency

1. Goblet cell dysfunctions : e.g. hypovitaminosis - A

2. Goblet cell distruction : e.g.

   - Alkali burn

   - Trachoma

   - Phemophigoid

   - Steven-Johnson syndrome

3. Drug induced :

   - Beta blockers (practolol)

   - Ecothiophate iodide

Causes of Aqueous-tear deficiency

1. Keratoconjunctivitis Sicca
2. Sjogren syndrome
3. Riley-Day syndrome
4. Trauma to lacrimal gland
5. Surgical removal of lacrimal gland
6. Infiltration by
   - Sarcoidosis
   - Lymphoma
     Amyloidosis
7. Drug induced
   - Antihistaminics
   - Antimuscarinics
   - Thiabendazole
8. Neoparalytic hyposecretion

WHO has classified defective vision into various grades :

Category of visual impairment	Best corrected visual acquity in the better eye	Interpretation	WHO Grade
0 (Normal)	6/6 to 6/18	Can see 6/18 or better	Normal
1 (Visual impairment)	<6/18 to 6/60	Cannot see 6/18 Can see 6/60	Low Vision (Category 1 & 2)
2 (Severe visual impairment)	<6/60 to 3/60	Cann see 6/60 Can see 3/60	
3	<3/60 to 1/60	Cannot see 3/60. Can see 1/60	Blindness (category 3,4 & 5)
4	<1/60 to only light perception	Cannot see 1/60 Can see light	
5	No light perception	Cannot see light.	
9			Unqualified visual loss

Note : Best corrected visual acquity of <6/60 to 3/60 in the better eye indicates severe visual impairment, but is also grouped into the category into the category of low vision.

Causes of Low Vision

Refractive Errors	**14.2%**
Cataract	7.6%
Trachoma	4.0%
Vitamin A deficiency	1.3%
Central corned opacity	0.7%
Trauma	0.07%

Major Intrinsic protein (MIP) of the lens is a 26k Da protein (MIP-26) that is exclusively expressed int he eye lens.

It belongs to the family of Aquaporins (Aquaporin O) and is involve in the transport of water across the lens.

MIP/Aquaporin 0 in the Eye lens

* Major intrinsic protein of the lens belongs to the super family of Aquaporins and is classified as Aqueoporin 0
* MIP 26 or Aquaproin 0 is permeable to water (water channels) and glycerol (glycerol channels).
* It serves two major functions to maintain the trnasparency of lens Transport of water across the lens
* Transport of glycerol across the lens.
* Aquaporin 0 or MIP mutations have been postulated to result formation of cataracts (loss of trnasparency of lens)

What important molecules constitute the interphoto receptor matrix?

1. Interphotoreceptor Retinal Binding Protein (IRBP)
2. Proteoglycans-Glycosaminoglycans
   * Sulphated/Non sulphated chondroitin
   * Hyaluronic Acid
3. Fibronectin
4. Sialoprotein associated with rods and cones (SPARC) (SPARC/Osteonectin/BM-40)
5. Intercellular Adhesion Molecule I (ICAM-1)
6. Hyaluronic Acid Receptor (CD44 antigen)
7. Lysosomal enzyme
   * Matrix metalloproteinases
   * Tissue Inhibitors of Metalloproteinases (TIMP)

Pathway for Horizontal Gaze

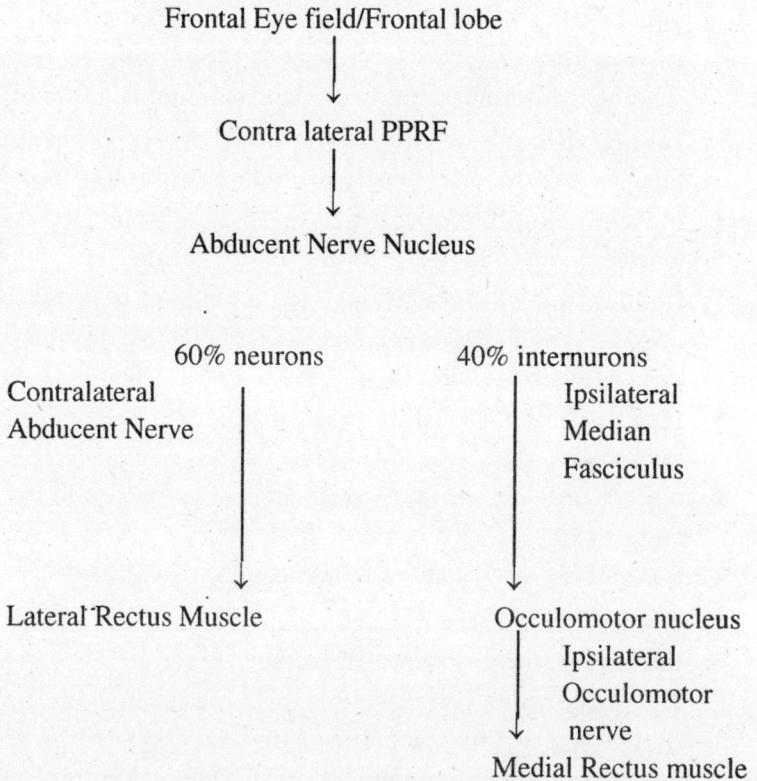

Frontal Eye field/Frontal lobe

↓

Contra lateral PPRF

↓

Abducent Nerve Nucleus

60% neurons	40% internurons
Contralateral Abducent Nerve	Ipsilateral Median Fasciculus
↓	↓
Lateral Rectus Muscle	Occulomotor nucleus
	Ipsilateral Occulomotor nerve
	↓
	Medial Rectus muscle

* In neurogenic ptosis, the amount of levator function is **inversely proportional** to the innervational defect.

* Blepharophimosis is inherited as an **autosomal dominant** trait.

* In congenital ptosis the ptotic lid is higher in down-gaze than the normal lid.

* Lid colobomas may be associated with dermoids.

* Atopic dermatitis may be associated with anterior subcapsular cataracts.

* A **blow out fracture** of the orbit may cause numbness of the upper lip.

* **Loss of vision** in the absence of significant proptosis may be seen in the Glioma of the optic nerve, apical cavernous haemangioma, apical granuloma, thyroid ophthalmopathy.

* **Enlargement** of the superior oribital fissure may be seen in infraclinoid aneurysms, intracavernous aneurysms, orbital tumours

* **Intraorbital calcification** is seen in orbital varices, optic nerve sheath meningiomas, lacrimal gland carcinoma, retinoblastoma.

* **Increased bone density** of the orbit is seen in meningioma, Paget's disease, osteoblastic secondaries, fibrous dysplasia.

* In **thyroid ophthalmopathy** an α-adrenergic blocking agent may be effective in the treatment of lid retraction.

* Bilateral **pseudotumour** may be associated with polyarteritis nodosa, Wedener's granulomatosis, Tuberculosis, Waldenstrom's macroglobulinaemia.

* Hand-Schuller-Christian disease is associated with diabetes insipidus.

* About 40% of children with neuroblastomas have orbital metastasis.

* Ewing's sarcoma cause a **haemorrhagic proptosis.**

* **Orbital metastasis** most commonly occurs from the bronchus, the kidney, the gastrointestinal tract,

* Disorders which may be associated with an aqueous deficiency of tears; psoriatic arthritis, Riley Day syndrome (familial dysautonomia), Pseudotumour, Hashimoto's thyroiditis, primary biliary cirrhosis.

* In **Sjogren's syndrome,** 50% have hypergammaglobulinaemia, 70-90% may be rheumatoid factor positive, 80% have antinuclear antibodies, anti DNA antibodies may be seen, antibodies to gastric parietal cells may be seen.

* The agents used in the tear substitutes are Polyethylene glycol 2%, Dextran 70.

* The iatrogenic causes of **punctal stenosis** .: IDU, Phospholine iodide, 5 FU.

* In investigation of the patency of the lacrimal drainage system, negative Jones-I test is indicative of a lacrimal pump failure.

* **Positive Jones-II test** is indicative of a partial nasolacrimal duct obstruction.

* Macrodacryocystography is useful to detect a filling defect caused by streptothrix.

* In nasolacrimal duct obstruction, involutional stenosis is probably the most common cause, Hydrostatic massage is effective in 95% of cases in the first year of life. Non-canalization at birth is frequent near the **valve of Hasner**. A DCR may be done for an incomplete obstruction.

* A mass usually below the medial canthal tendon may be indicative of a lacrimal sac tumour.

* **Canaliculitis** is commonly caused by herpes simplex infection.

* A mucocele is an indication for a DCR.

* Blepharitis may be associated with the following signs on the lid margin : Madarosis, Poliosis, Trichiasis, Collarettes, Rosettes (dilated blood vessels).

* Ophthalmia neonatorum may be caused by herpes simplex.

* Spring catarrh may give rise to trantas dots, corneal plaques, cupid's bow.

* Superior limbic keratoconjunctivitis (SLK) is more common in woman. SLK is associated with dysthyroid eye disease.

* Hutchinson's freckle is **precancerous**.

* **Goldenhar's syndrome** may be associated with Choriostomas, Hemifacial hypoplasia, Strabismus, Optic nerve hypoplasia, Tilted disc.

* In the cornea, the Bowman's membrane is acellular.

* Filamentary keratitis may be seen in prolonged patching of the eyelid, superior limbic keratoconjunctivitis, herpes zoster, Sjogren's syndrome.

* Gross pannus formation may be seen in Rosacea, Pemphigoid.

* **Melanin** and **Krukenberg's spindle** are associated.

* Brolene and neomycin are effective in **amoebic keratitis.**

* **Cogan's syndrome** may be associated with polyarteritis nodosa.

* Herpetic eye disease may be precipitated by systemic corticosteroids, trauma, sunshine, psychiatric disturbances.

* In primary herpes simplex infections of the eye, pre-auricular adenopathy is seen, 50% develop a keratitis, disciform keratitis is rare.

* Pseudodendrites are associated with soft contact lens wear, healing corneal abrasions.

* Decreased corneal sensation occurs in diabetes, Riley-Day syndrome, Lattice corneal dystrophy, Anhidrotic ectodermal dysplasia.

* In peripheral corneal ulcerations, Contact lens cornea may be associated with rheumatoid arthritis.

* **Salzmann's nodular degeneration** in cornea occurs following trachoma.

* Fuchs endothelial dystrophy is **autosomal dominant.**

* Cornea verticillata may be associated with or seen in the treatment of systemic lupus erythematosis, cardiac arrythmias, α-Galactosidase-A deficiency, breast carcinoma, arthritis.

* Corneal depositions are associated with the mucopolysaccharidosis Morquio's.

* Hard lenses are usually small and steep.

* **Radial keratotomy** may be followed by diurnal fluctuations of vision.

* **Epikeratophakia** may be used to treat Aphakia, myopia, keratoconus, hypermetropia.

* In uveitis, **floaters** are usually the presenting feature of pars planitis, associated with sarcoidosis, development of disc new vessels may be a feature.

* **Masquerade syndromes** include melanoma, histiocytic lymphoma.

* In the uveitis associated with juvenile chronic arthritis the eye is white even in the presence of severe uveitis, the second eye involvement in unilateral cases is rare after one year.

* In the uveitis associated with juvenile chronic arthritis. The eye is white even in the presence of severe uveitis, the second eye involvement in unilateral cases is rare after one year.

* **Vogt-Koyanagi-Harada syndrome** affects the posterior segment initially as a multifocal choroiditis.

* The drugs used in the treatment of vision-threatening toxoplasmosis : Clindamycin, Pyrimethamine,.

* In ocular manifestations of acquired immunodeficiency syndrome (AIDS) : **CMV retinitis** is a major cause of visual loss, 50% of patients have transient cotton wool spots; Skin tumours of the lids are a feature, scattered retinal nerve fibre haemorrhage can occur as in isolated feature.

* Presumed ocular histoplasmosis is characterized by **Histot spots,** peripapillary atrophy, Haemorrhagic disciform macular degeneration.

* Heterochromic cyclitis has small stellate KPs scattered all over the cornea as a **pathognomonic feature.**

* The cytotoxic agent used in uveitis is Azathioprine.

* Pigmentation of the trabecular meshwork is more prominent inferiorly in Trauma, Uveitis, Pseudoexfoliation, Senile eyes.

* Blood in the Schlemm's canal is commonly seen in Sturge—Weber syndrome, Hypotony, Caroticocavernous fistula.

* Blood vessels may be observed in the angle in normal eyes, in chronic uveitis, as a complication of diabetes, and glaucoma.

* **Kinetic perimetry** may be performed on a Lister's perimeter.

* In the management of primary open angle glaucoma (POAG) with miotics, Iris cysts may be prevented by concomitant use of phenylephrine.

* The side effects of dichlorphenamide include depression, decreased libido, renal stones, metabolic acidosis, Stevens-hohnson syndrome.

* Following Argon laser trabeculoplasty, **transient** pressure elevations occur in 25% of cases. The pressure rise is commonly detected within the **first three hours,** anterior non-granulomatous uveitis is seen, permanent intraocular pressure elevations occur in 3% of cases.

* Excellent result with argon laser trabeculoplasty occur in Glaucoma capsulare, eyes with primary open angle glaucoma prior to lens extraction, Pigmentary glaucoma.

* Argon laser iridotomy causes less bleeding, failure of iridotomy patency is commoner with argon laser.

* In pigment dispersion syndrome, the size and density of the Krukenberg spindle is **directly proportional** to the extent of associated iris atrophy, extreme retinal periphery may have pigment deposition.

* The **pseudoexfoliation syndrome** causes glaucoma in 60% of affected eyes, with a hyperpigmented trabecular meshwork.

* In the formation of a cataract and its morphology, Galactokinase deficiency is responsible for some forms of presenile cataract.

* α-Galactosidase deficiency is associated with **spokelike lens opacities,** α-2-Globulin deficiency is associated with **sunflower cataract.**

* In systemic diseases associated with cataract, hypoparathyroidism is associated with small white flecks of cataract which rarely progress to maturity.

* The posterior subcapsular lens opacities are seen in gyrate atrophy of the retina, Stickler's syndrome, Leber's congenital amaurosis.

* In the evaluation of congenital cataracts, bilateral cataracts have a more favourable visual outcome than unilateral cataracts. Delayed treatment of unilateral cataract leads to structural changes in the geniculocortical pathways.

* Abnormal vitreoretinal adhesions are noted at the posterior border of lattice degeneration, areas of white without pressure, congenital cystic retinal tufts.

* The dome-shaped **mirror of the Goldman** allows visualization of ora serrata.

* Snail track degeneration has the same complications as lattice degeneration.

* **Giant tears** are associated with areas of white without pressure.

* **Snow flake degeneration** is important because it is frequently associated with other vitreoretinal degenerations of importance.

* In the surgical management of retinal detachment, inferior equatorial tears require subretinal fluid drainage, air may be used to flatten radial retinal folds.

* Features that suggest **preproliferative diabetic retinopathy** include : large blot haemorrhages, intraretinal microvascular anomalies, **'Sausage-like'** segmentation of veins, arteriolar narrowing.

* In proliferative diabetic retinopathy : It has been estimated that one-quarter of the retina has to be non-perfused before new vessels develop, the predilection of new vessels on the disc is due to the absence of an internal limiting membrane, total vitreous detachment could lead to a regression of new vessels, vitreous haemorrhage may be precipitated by severe physical exertion, pregnancy may adversely affect on this stage of eye disease.

* In proliferative diabetic retinopathy : NVD have a **greater propensity to bleed** than NVE. NVE without vitreous haemorrhage untreated have a 10% chance of severe visual loss in two years, NVE without vitreous haemorrhage have a 7% risk of severe visual loss in two years. A sign of involution of new vessels after PRP is pallor of the optic disc.

* In the treatment of vitreous haemorrhage in proliferative diabetic retinopathy, in the absence of rubeosis irides and vitreous haemorrhage early victrectomy should be considered in insulin dependent patient, associated with rubeosis irides, early vitrectomy allows PRP which prevents neovascular glaucoma.

* Recognized **risk factors** in the development of central retinal vein occlusion are : Waldenstrom's macroglobulinaemia, Behcet's disease.

* Retinal artery occlusion is associated with mural thrombus, atrial myxoma, scleroderma, myocarditis, angle closur glaucoma.

* In the pathogenesis and clinical feature of retinopathy of prematurity (ROP), vascularization of the retina starts at the fourth month of gestation, plus disease is characterized by venous dilation and tortuosity of the arterioles, myopia is a feature of cicatricial disease.

* In the macula area, the internal limiting membrane is **thinnest** within the fovea.

* Subretinal neovascular membranes are associated with Serpiginous choriodopathy, rubella retinopathy, Best's disease, excessive photocoagulation.

* Central serous chorioretinopathy manifests as an acquired hypermetropia.

* **Lacquer cracks** have a predilection of fundi of highly myopic young adults, macular pucker is a complication of retinal, **choroidal folds** may occur for no apparent reason bilaterally in hypermetropic patients with normal vision.

* **Angioid streaks** are associated with optic nerve head drusen, Groenblad-Strandberg syndrome, sickle cell disease.

* **Bulls eye maculopathy** may occur during treatment of malaria in non-endemic areas, systemic lupus erythematosus (SLE)

* In the electroretinogram : The 'β' wave arises from the retinal pigment epithelium. The 'β' wave is generated by the **Muller cells.**

* The inheritance of **retinitis pigmentosa** is autosomal dominant, autosomal recessive, X-linked recessive.

* Retinitis pigmentosa is associated with Translucent vitreous floaters, optic nerve head drusen, cellophane maculopathy, myopia.

* Systemic associations of retinitis pigmentosa include Ataxia, acanthocytosis, heart block, non-progressive sensorineural deafness, malabsorption.

* Luber's congenital amaurosis is associated with oculodigital syndrome, keratoconus, renal abnormalities, epilepsy.

* **Best's disease** is associated with a subretinal neovascular membrane in stage V of the disease.

* **Cherry red spot** at the macula is identified in infantile amaurotic familial idiocy, GM2 gangliosidosis type 2, Niemann-Pick disease, Sialidosis.

* The ERG and EOG are **normal** in central areolar choroidal dystrophy, Wagener's disease.

* An iris melanoma is usually composed of spindle cells.

* Retinoblastoma which is associated with abundant rosettes histopathologically has a **poorer prognosis** than a retinoblastoma with none.

* Spontaneous hyphaema may occur in Retinoblastoma, Juvenile xanthogranuloma, Incontinentia pigmenti.

* The following are recognized clinical features of persistent hyperplastic primary vitreous : Elongated ciliary processes, cataract, angle closure glaucoma, microphthalmia.

* A horopter is an imaginary surface in space all points of which still stimulate corresponding retinal elements and are therefore projected to the same position in space, **Pannum's area** is a zone surrounding points on the horopter in which objects are seen singly.

* In evaluation of diplopia **Hess chart** may be used as a prognostic guide to recovery.

* **Hirschberg's test** is useful in eliminating pseudostrabismus, a 4 diopters prism in front of a squinting eye (with microtropia) does not include corrective movement.

* Infantile (congenital) esotropia is associated with cerebral palsy.

* In non-refractive accommodative esotropia bimedial recession is the surgical procedure of choice,

* The helpful methods in the treatment of amblyopia are Pleoptics, Cam therapy, Occlusion, Penalization.

* **Duane's retraction syndrome** is congenital, is associated with co-contraction of the horizontal recti, may be associated with congenital skeletal defects.

* **Mobius syndrome** has the following clinical features : Infantile feeding difficulties, exposure keratitis, atrophy of the tongue, and expressionless face.

* In the surgical correction of ocular motility disorders 'A' pattern esotropia is treated by bilateral medial rectus recession with upward transposition. **Faden procedure** is used to correct DVD, **Hummelsheim procedure** is used for correction of sixth nerve palsy, adjustable sutures are used for surgery in cases of thyroid myopathy.

* Arcuate defects in the visual field may occur in optic nerve head drusen, Optic neuritis, optic neuropathy (ischaemic), optic nerve head cupping.

* In multiple sclerosis with optic neuritis, colour vision is severely impaired even in patients with relatively good visual acuity.

* Anterior ischaemic optic neuropathy occurs in Polyarteritis nodosa, migraine, atherosclerosis, giant cell arteritis, papilloedema.

* In optic nerve gliomas, diffuse enlargement of the optic foramina are noted on the Rhese View X-ray.

* In diabetes, the pupil is **spared.**

* **Painful ophthalmoplegia** is caued by Tolosa-Hunt syndrome, Diabetes, Aneurysms.

* **Light near dissociation** may occur in Juvenile diabetes, aberrant regeneration of the third nerve, pinealomas, neurosyphilis, dystrophia myotonica.

* Congenital nystagmus may be dampened by convergence.

* The bony orbit is a pear-shaped cavity that is made from constituents of **seven** individual bones.

* All paranasal sinuses are normally present at birth (apart from the frontal sinus which is rudimentary until **2 years** of age). All sinuses are lined by pseudostratified columnar ciliated epithelium.

* The embryonic nucleus is the **innermost** nucleus of the lens.

* Muller cells are responsible for the nutrition of retinal resources, and are responsible for the β wave of the electroetinogram.

* The central retinal artery arises from the ophthalmic artery where it lies **inferolateral** to the optic nerve.

* *Staphylococcus epidermidis* is found in up to 70% of eyes, and *Staphylococcus aureus in* approximately 45°. The most common anaerobe is *Propionibacterium acnes.*

* Protozoan commensals include *Demodex follicularum* (found on the eye lashes in almost everyone over 70 years of age). Up to 100 fungi (including *Pityrosporon orbiculari,* a yeast found on the lasthes and lid margins) have been found.

* **Cottonwool spots** are the most common findings in AIDS.

* *Candida albicans* can also cause a retinitis whose appearance is often mistaken for that of the cottonwool spots induced by ischaemia.

* ELISA is the **most sensitive** and **specific diagnostic** aid for toxocariasis.

* The chance of congenital toxoplasmosis is increased if the maternal infection is in the third trimester, but the severity of the illness is **greatest** if the infection occurs in the first **trimester**.

* **Flucytosine** has a limited spectrum, including candidiasis or cryptococcosis.

* **Foscarnet** appears to be about as effective as gancicyovir for the initial **2-3 weeks** induction therapy of CMV retinitis.

* **Type-II MHC** antigens are classified by HLA D sequences, and are found predominantly on macrophages, Langhans cells, dendritic cells, and occasionally on cells that have been exposed to gamma interferon.

* The ideal topical preparation should be biphasic so that it can pass through the hydrophilic and hydrophobic layers of the cornea.

* The only known ocular side effect of phenytoin is nystagmus.

* The protein content of the lens is higher than in any other body tissue (33% of lens weight). Soluble proteins such as α, β and γ crystallins make up 85% of the total protein content. β Crystallines accounts for 50% of these soluble proteins; a crystalline is predominantly found in the cortex.

* Lipids account for 5% of the dry weight of the lens (cholesterol approximately 50%, phospholipid 45%, glycosphingolipids 5%), and the cholesterol) phospholipid ratio is higher than in any other tissue. Glycolysis utilises 80% of the lens glucose but does not produce a correspondingly high percentage of the ATP output as glycolysis will produce a net gain of only **2 ATP** for every glucose molecule.

* The **near triad** consists of convergence, accommodation and pupillary constriction (not dilatation).

* The framework of the vitreous is made up of specialised type of collagen called **vitrosin.**

* **Anisocoria** is increased in dim light because the normal pupil will dilate, whereas the Horner's pupil will not.

* The exact details of the critical period for acquity in humans are not as well as defined those for experimental animals.

* **Optotypes** all derive from the Landholdt "C".

* Tear film is composed of 3 layers: a **lipid layer** (by tarsal glands), second **aqueous layer** (from glands of Krause & Wolfring) and inner **hydrophilic mucin layer** (by goblet cells), is 0.05 mm thick.

* **CONTRIBUTORS TO OPHTHALMOLOGY :**

1. **Hippel's :** (*Eugen von Hippel*)
   * Disease
   * Operation

2. **Horner's** (*Willian Edmunds Horner*)
   * Law
   * Muscle
   * Ptosis
   * Pupil
   * Syndrome (Oculo-pupillary)

3. **Hutchinson's :** *Sir Jonathan Hutchinson*)
   * Facies
   * Pupil
   * Teeth
   * Triad
   * Syndrome

4. **Imre's :** (*Josef Imre*)
   * Operation (to close lid defects)
   * Treatment

5. **Ishihara's :** (*Shinobu Ishihara*)
   * Plate
   * Test (for colour vision)

6. **Jensen's :** (*Edmund Zeuthen Jensen*)
   * Disease
   * Retinitis

7. **Kimmelstiel-Wilson :**
   * Disease
   * Syndrome

8. **Kayser & Richard Fleischer :**
   * Kayser-Fleischer corneal ring

9. **Koeppe's :**
   * Disease
   * Nodule

10. **Krause's :** (*Carl Fiedric Thodre Krauser*)
    * Gland (Accessory-lacrimal)
    * Syndrome

11. **Kuhnt's :**
    * Forceps
    * Illusion
    * Operation

12. **Landolt's :**
    * Bodies
    * Operation

13. **Laurenc-Moon-Biedl :** *(John Zachariah Laurence Robert H. Moon & Arthur Beidl)*
    * Syndrome
14. **Leber's :** *(Theodore L. Leber)*
    * Amaurosis
    * Disease
15. **Lowe's**
    * Ring
    * Syndrome
16. **Maddox :**
    * Prism
    * Rod
    * Wing
17. **Marfan's :** *(Bernard-Jean Antonin Marfan)*
    * Syndrome
18. **Maxwell's**
    * Ring
    * Spot
19. **Meibom :** *(Heinrich Meibom)*
    * Cyst
    * Glands
20. **Mikulicz's :** *(Johann von Mikulicz Radecki)*
    * Disease
    * Syndrome
21. **Millard-Gubler :** *(August L.J. Millard & A. Gubler)*
    * Syndrome
22. **Morgagnian :** *(Giovanni Battista Morgagni)*
    * Cataract
23. **Mobius :**
    * Disease
    * Sign
    * Syndrome
24. **Muller's :**
    * Fibres (sustentacular)
    * Muscle (Circular cillary & plain muscle)
    * Trigone
25. **Q' Brien's :**
    * Akinesia
    * Block
    * Cataract
    * Forceps
26. **Parinaud's :** *(Henri Parinaud)*
    * Conjunctivitis
    * Ophthalmoplegia
    * Syndrome
27. **Pick's :**
    * Retinitis
    * Vision
28. **von Recklinghausen's :** *(Friedrich Daniel von Recklinghausen)*
    * Disease
    * Lymph canals (of Recklinghausen in cornea)
29. **Argyll Robertson :** *(Douglas Murray Cooper Lamb Argyll Robertson)*
    * Pupil

30. **Louis Joseph Sanson & Johannes Evangelista Purkinje :**
    * Purkinje Sanson image
31. **Schiotz :** *(Hajalmar Schiotz)*
    * Tonometer
32. **Schlemm :** *(Friedrichs Schlemm)*
    * Canal of Schlemm
33. **Schnabel's :** *(Isidor Schnabel)*
    * Optic atrophy
34. **Seidel's :** *(Erich Seidel)*
    * Sign (Scotoma)
35. **Sjogren's :**
    * Disease
    * Syndrome
36. **Snellen's :** *(Henry Snellen)*
    * Chart
    * Implant
    * Operation
    * Reform eye
37. **Soemmering's :**
    * Ring
    * Spot
38. **Stellwag's :**
    * Brawny edema
    * Sign
39. **Sturge-Weber :** *(William Allen Sturge and Fredrick Parkes Weber)*
    * Syndrome (Neuro-cutaneous)

40. **Tay's :** *(Waren Tay)*
    * Choroiditis (Central guttate)
    * Spot or dots or colloid bodies
41. **Tenon's** (Jacques Rene Tenon)
    * Capsule
    * Episcleral tissue
    * Fascia
    * Space
42. **Troutman's :**
    * Implant
    * Operation
43. **Van Lint :**
    * Akinesia
    * Block
    * Technique
44. **Vossius's :** *(Adolf Vossius)*
    * Lenticular ring opacity
45. **Vogt's :** *(Alfred Vogt)*
    * Cataract
    * Cornea
    * Degeneration
    * Disease
    * Syndrome
46. **von Graefe's :**
    * Cautery
    * Cystotome
    * Forceps
    * Hook
    * Knife

* Knife needle
* Operation
* Sign

47. **Weber's** : *(Sir Hermann Weber)*
    * Knife
    * Sign
    * Syndrome

48. **Week's** *(John Elmer Weeks)*
    * Bacillus *(Haemophilus influenzae)*
    * Needle
    * Operation
    * Speculum

49. **Westphal's** : *(Alexander Karl Otto Westphal)*
    * Reaction

50. **Wilder's** : *(William Wilder)*
    * Scoop
    * Sign

51. **Wilson** : *(Samuel Alexander Kinnier Wilson)*
    * Hepatolenticular degeneration
    * Disease (Kinnier-Wilson's disease)

52. **Zinn's** : *(John Gottfried Zinn)*
    * Circlet arteriosis
    * Corona
    * Ligaments (Annulus & Suspensory)
    * Tendon
    * Zonule

HISTORY

* 600 B.C. **Sushruta**—First ancient ophthalmic surgeon, devised first cataract operation and pterygium operation.

* 1452 **Leonardo da Vinci**—Studied ocular anatomy, described pupillary reaction to light and recognised retina as organ of vision.

* **Bangerter**—First advocated the use of pleoptics.

* 1579-1650 **Cristopher Scheiner**—Made the first measurement of corneal curvature.

* 1621 **Willebaord Snell**—Formulated the laws of reflection and refraction.

* 1752 **Daviel Jacques**—Performed first operation of extraction of cataract and devised Daviel's scoop or spoon.

* 1773 **Thomas Young**—Described astigmatism, theory of colour vision, theory of accommodation and mapped normal field of vision.

* 1775 **Benjamin Franklin**—Made the first bifocal spectacle lens.

* 1809-1852 **Louis Braille**—Devised a system of embossed printing or writing for the blind (Braille system) — himself sightless.

* 1827 **Sir George Biddell Airy**—Corrected his own astigmatism.

* 1831 **Holmgren**—Discovered electroretinogram (ERG) and test for colour vision (Holmgren's test)

* **Filatov**—Pioneered the use of cadaver eyes for corneal transplantation.

* 1851 **Hermann von Helmholtz**—Invented the direct ophthalmoscope (**Young-Helmholtz**)—has propounded the trichromatic theory of colour irregular astigmatism.

* **Harold Ridley**—Began using PMMA intraocular lens implantation.

* 1954, **Goldmann**—Devised applantation tonometer, gonioscopy on slit lamp and gonio-lens and contact lens for fundus examination.

* **Otoo Wichterle**—Introduced a soft hydrophilic plastic and made the first soft contact lens.

* **Bergmeister's papilla**—A small mass (embryological) of glial cells that surrounds the hyaloid artery in the centre of the optic disc (persists in adult eye).

* **Cloquet's canal** is space in the vitreous (formerly contained the hyaloid artery during development).

* **Hassall-Henle warts**—Excrescences or thickenings of Descemet's membrane (occur as a normal aging change in the peripheral cornea).

* **Mittendorf dot**—Opacity of the posterior lens capsule (marking the former site of congenital hyaloid artery attachment).

* **Meyer's loop**—The most anterior inferior fibres of the optic radiation from Meyer's loop.

* **'Venae Vorticosae'** are the most important (open into ophthalmic vein) in draining the uveal tract.

* **Vitreous** has no blood vessels & it derives nutrition from the surrounding structures (choroid, ciliary body & retina).

* **Glass Rod-Phenomenon :**
  * **Blood influx into the aqueous vein**—Occurs during a rising phase of tension in Glaucoma & Paracentesis.
  * **Aqueous influx into the blood vein**—Seen in a falling phase or when external pressure is put upon the globe.
* The hyaloid system atrophies completely by the eighth month.
* The aqueous drainage system is ready to function before birth.
* The pupillary reflexes appear at about the **fifth fetal month** and are active by the **sixth month.**
* The lids develops from mesoderm except for the skin and conjunctiva.
* The main function of sclera is protective.
* Stercopsis is a higher quality of binocular vision.
* Rods & cones are the end-organs of vision.
* **Phagosomes** are known to be discarded rod discs that have been engulfed by the pigment epithelium.
* Lateral wall is the thickest wall of bony orbit where as medial wall is the thinnest one.
* Excrescences or thickenings of Descemet's membrane may occur as a normal aging change in the peripheral cornea (**Hassall-Henle warts**) and are considered abnormal when they occur in the central cornea (**corneal guttata).**
* The use of red glasses, dark rooms, and X-ray rooms permit individuals to maintain full cone function while the rods become dark adapted.
* The venae vorticosae drain into both superior and inferior ophthalmic veins.
* **Endoderm** does not contribute to the formation of the eye.
* At birth, the eye is larger in relation to the rest of the body (than in the case of children & adults).
* At birth, the lens is more nearly spherical in shape than later in life.
* The lens grows throughout life as new fibres are added to the periphery, making it flatter.

* When the iris is cut (as in small peripheral iridectomy) it seldom bleeds and the wound remains permanently with no tendency to heal.

* Hyaloid canal is otherwise known as **Cloquet's canal.**

* Macula lutea nourishment is entirely dependent upon the choroid.

* Most of the orbital veins drain into the superior ophthalmic vein.

* The longest extra-ocular muscle is superior oblique muscle.

* The posterior end of inferior oblique muscle insertion is almost overlies the macula.

* The eyeball occupies only about one-fifth of the volume of the orbit and is situated anteriorly in the orbit, just within the protective orbital margin.

* **Plica semilunaris** (small crescentric fold of conjunctiva) is a vestigial structure homologus with a nictitating membrane.

* The vitreous body comprises **two thirds** of the volume of the eye.

* Tear production is decreased during the night.

* Highest venous pressure in the body is in episcleral veins.

* The avascular structures of eye are cornea, lens, vitreous and macula.

* The fetal lens is spherical.

* **Fovea centralis has—**
  * No rods (but has only cones).
  * No direct blood vessels.
  * No nerve fibre layer.
  * Scotopic vision is the function of rods.
  * Optic disc is the blind spot of Mariotte.

* **Circulus arteriosus iridis major** is situated in the anterior part of the ciliary body at the base of the iris where as **Circulus arteriosus iridis minor** is situated at a little outside the pupillary margin.

* Lens has highest protein content of any tissue of the body

* The only blood supply to the fovea centralis (susceptible to irrepairable damage when the retina is detached) is **Chorio-capillaries.**

* The retina has no pain nerve fibre.
* Aqueous in the aphakic eye contains more glucose than in normal eye.
* **Fermat's principle**—A ray of light passing from one point to another follows the path that takes the least time to negotiate.
* **Strum's internal or conoid of Strum**—Geometric representation of light refracted through a lens that is spherical along one axis and cylindrical along another (It consists of two focal lines separated by the interval of Strum).
* **Schematic eye of Gullstrand**—It is a data for distance of the cardinal point from anterior surface of cornea and from these data the refractive.
* **Sanders-Retziaff-Kraf or SRK equation**—Determines the necessary intraocular lens power as follows :

  Power of IOL=A-2.5 L - 0.9 K

  A = Constant for the particular lens

  K = Average keratometer readings

  L = Axial length in millimeters
* **Fogging**—A method of determine refractive error in which accommodation is relaxed (by means of convex spheres) and that make the patient artificially myopic.
* **Pseudophakia**—Implanted artifical intraocular lens implant following cataract extractions.
* **Theories of light**—Particle theory (Plank) and wave theory (Maxwell).
* **Descartes' law**—See Snell's law on next page.
* **Donders' law**—Every oblique position of the eyeball is associated with a constant amount of torsional movement.
* **Flouren's law**—Stimulation of a semicircular canal results in nystagmus in the plane of that canal.
* **Hering's law**—
  1. The distinctness of a sensation depends on the relation between its intensity and the total intensity of all simultaneous sensation.

2. Any central stimulation, whether excitatory or inhibitory, reaches both eyes equally, so that movement of the two eyes is independent but takes place in the same direction to the same extent.

* **Horner's law**—Colour blindness is transmitted from the male through an unaffected female to the male, i.e. sex-linked recessive transmission.

* **Listing's law**—When the line of fixation of the eye passes from its primary position to any other position, the angle of torsion of the eye in this second position is the same as if the eye had arrived at this position by turning about a fixed axis perpendicular to the initial and final positions of the line of fixation.

* **Sherrington's law**—The eyes are maintained in the primary position, by a state of slight contraction or tonus of all the extra-ocular muscles. (When any movement takes place, some muscles relax and others contract).

* **Snell's law**—A ray of light which passes from one medium to another, the sine of the angle of incidence bears a ratio to the sine of the angle of refraction that is a constant for the two given media.

* **Others laws include :**
  * Desmarres's law
  * Ewald's law
  * Giraud-Teulon law
  * Gullstrand's law

* **Gaussian frequency curve** will have a certain skew deviation at birth.

* By far the **commonest** cause of defective visual acuity is a refractive error.

* Spectacles - frames are now most commonly made of **Cellulose acetate** (a thermoplastic).

* Myopia must never be over corrected.

* Presbyopic spectacles should never be prescribed mechanically by ordering an approximate addition varying with the age of the patient.

* Curvature myopia occurs commonly as a factor in astigmatism.

* **Index myopia** accounts for myopia of senile cataract due to ↑ in refractive index of the nucleus of the lens.

* The **most powerful** refracting surface of the eye is front surface of the cornea.
* The only symptom in low myopia may be indistinct distant vision.
* The newborn are almost invariably hypermetropic (average 2.5 D).
* The retinal image of the aphakic eye is about a quarter larger than the emmetropic retinal image.
* Pathological curvature myopia is seen typically in conical cornea.
* The anterior lens capsule is responsible for functional accommodation.
* Prisms are used diagnostically to assess the type and magnitude of a strabismus and to treat diplopia.
* The two most important differential diagnosis for high hyperopia and high myopia are **pseudooptic neuritis** (with elevated & blurred nerve head) and **unilateral exophthalmous** respectively.
* The instrument used to measure aniseikonia is called an **eikonometer,** and aniseikonia is corrected by lenses known as **isokonic (iseikonic) lenses.**
* Test for measuring phorias include cover-unocver test, Maddox wing and von Graefe test, Duane test or cover test.
* The power of a lens depends on its refractive index and its curvature.
* Curvature myopia occurs commonly as a factor in astigmatism.
* In degenerative axial myopia, the increase in length of the eye affects the posterior poles and the surrounding area.
* Retinoscopy is done at a distance of one metre.
* Visual angle is the angle substended by the object at the nodal point.
* The suitable agent to dilate pupil in hypermetropoic eyes of children is atropine.
* Radial keratotomy is an operative treatment for myopia.
* The anatomic factor causing strongest correlation with refraction is axial length of the eye ball.
* The fair point or punctum remotum is virtual in hypermetropia.

* The punctum proximum of the eye varies according to its static refraction and the age of patient.

* The standard power of an IOL, implanted in posterior chamber in an emetropic eye is **20 diopters.**

* Removal of crystalline lens surgically may be advocated in high myopia.

* Occasional intoleration of bifocal lens may be due to chromatic aberration, prismatic jump, lack of intermediate focus and muscle imbalance.

* Concave mirror retinoscopy is useful in a patient with haze media and with high degree of ametropia.

* The subjective varification of refractive error may be done by astigmatic fan and cross-cylinder.

* Foster-Fuchs spots may be the complication of myopia.

* Telescopic spectacles help in magnification of words in retinal disease.

* The refractometer assesses the degree of ametropia.

* The basic principles of stenopeic slit is **pinhole phenomenon.**

* The most accepted aetiological theory of myopia is that is due to strongly hereditary and genetically predetermined.

* In streak retinoscopy, the streak effect is obtained by using plano-cylindrical retinoscopy mirror.

* In young children, hypermetropia is a predisposing cause of convergent strabismus.

* All accommodation is lost in Aphakia.

* Contact lenses will not eliminate all the visual field anomalies of aphakia.

* S,G,H and B are the **easiest** letters to recognize on the Snellen chart, where as L,T,U,V and C are the five most difficult ones.

* Rays between 600 mμ and 295 mμ reach the lens, those between 400 mμ & 350 mμ can reach retina of normal eye and between 400 mμ & 295 mμ can reach retina of lensless eye.

* The pigment epithelium on the back of the iris and the retinal pigmentary epithelium at the back of the eye absorb radiation of all wavelengths.

* Concave mirror is used in the ordinary use of ophthalmic instruments.
* Highly hypermetropic eyes are smaller than normal.
* **Dynamic retinoscopy** gives an objective basis of refraction of the eye for near vision.
* The eye is normally myopic for blue rays and eye is normally hypermetropic for red rays.
* In presbyopia it is better that the condition is under corrected.
* After removal of lens the eye becomes highly hypermetropic.
* Image jump occurs with the use of bifocal lens.
* A **lensometer** is used to measure the equivalent power of the lens.
* In subjective verification of the refraction cross cylinder helps in establishing both the power and axis of the cylinder.
* The manifestation of presbyopia in hypermetropia occurs at an earlier age than usual.
* The greatest incidence of severe microbial keratitis is found in patients wearing soft contact lens.
* Myopes have larger pupils than hyperopes.
* The ciliary muscle contraction can only correct hypermetropia.
* Pseudopapillitis is seen in hypermetropia.
* Distant vision is often found to be surprisingly good with mixed astigmatism.
* Asthenopia caused by astigmatism is often worse with lower degree of astigmatism.
* Fuchs fleck is seen in degenerative myopia.
* Strum's conoid phenominon tell about curvature ametropia.
* Hyperopia is a frequenty cause of oestropia and monocular amblyopia.
* Ophthalmoscopically the fundus may exhibit no abnormality in hypermetropia.
* Anisometropia may cause asthenopic symptoms.
* Refractive errors are inherited.
* The principle of the stenopic slit is based on **Pinhole phenomenon.**

* **'Jack-in-the Box'** ring scotoma from prismatic effects at the edge of the spectacle lens occurs an **Aphakic eye.**

* **Telescopic spectacles** may provide sufficient magnification to permit reading in visual failure due to retinal disease.

* Aniseikonia (different image size in each eye) is measured with **Goldmann eikonometer.**

* Base curves of lenses can be checked with a **Geneva lens measure.**

* Simple myopia usually becomes apparent at about the age of **Eight years.**

* Geometric representation of light refracted through a lens that is spherical along an axis and cylindrical along another is known as **Strum's conoid.**

* Old age hypermetropia is due to index hypermetropia.

* **Examination of Recess of angle of AC :**
  * *Gonioscopy*—to visualise recess of the angle of AC.
  * *Direct Gonioscope*—Keoppes, Barkans & Worst.
  * *Indirect Gonioscope*—Goldmann (3 mirror), Zeis 14 mirror & Allenthorpes.

* *Normal structures visualise through Gonioscope include :*
  * Anterior surface of cornea
  * Antero-medial surface of ciliary body
  * Trabecular meshwork
  * Schwalbe's line
  * Posterior surface of cornea

* **Alcian blue dye**—Stains mucus selectivity and delineates excess mucus produced when there is a difficulty in tear formation.

* Grey iris with ill defined pattern—> atrophy from cyclitis or glaucoma.

* Darkly pigmented spots (not raised)—> Normal iris (**differential diagnosis :** Brown/Grey raised nodules, melanoma, tubercle, gumma).

* Muddiness of Iris—>inflammatory exudative iritis.

* **Agar triad**—Aniridia, genitourinary abnormalities and mental retardation.
* **Babbage** invented ophthalmoscopy.
* von Helm Holtz reinvented its importance.
* Rente introduced the perforated concave mirror in place of plane mirror.
* Fluorescein ocular stain becomes easily contaminated with **Pseudomonas aeruginosa.**
* Cleaning of the tonometer to prevent AIDS include H_2O_2 **and Tono film** (disposable rubber cap—an excellent device).
* Before instilling the mydriatic, examine the anterior chamber by oblique illumination with a hand light.
* In any patient over 20 years of age, tonometry should be performed as a screening test for glaucoma.
* With a slit lamp without any additional aid one can examine upto anterior vitreous.
* Colour perimetry is useful in the diagnosis of retrobulbar neuritis.
* Rose Bengal stains are for —diseased and devitalized cells.
* The aqueous flare is best seen by **Biomicroscope.**
* One entering the blood stream fluorescein dye is readily bound to albumin.
* The darker colour of the macula is due to the presence of **luteal pigment.**
* In an eye with opaque ocular media the retinal detachment can be diagnosed by **ocular ultrasonography.**
* **Electro-oculography (EOG)** denotes the health of pigment epithelial cells and outer segment of visual receptors.
* "All red eyes are not pink eyes".
* The Ishihara plates can only identify defects in red-green discrimination, whereas the American Optical Hardy-Rand-Rittler (HRR) plates are useful in detecting red-green and blue yellow defects.
* Colour vision should be tested separately with each eye (optic neuritis may be responsible for a monocular type of acquired colour defect).

* In physical examination of the eye, by far the most important single examination is visual acuity testing in each eye.

* Determining the intraocular pressure by finger palpation of the eye (tactile tension) is not a reliable procedure.

* The troublesome reflexes formed by the surface of the lens and the eye in indirect ophthalmoscopy are checked by slightly tilting the lens.

* For measuring the axial length of the eye ball, best pulse **A scan echo technique on ultrasonography** is useful.

* The fundus background is tigroid or tesselated if the pigment is deficient in retinal pigment epithelium.

* **Photostress test** is useful in early macular disease.

* Normally, pulsations seen on the optic disc are venous pulsations.

* Phototopic ERG or foveal ERG is helpful in diagnosing macular degeneration in the presence of cataract.

* Gross intraocular haemorrhage gives no external ocular sign.

* A corrected visual acuity of less than 6/9 (20/30) is abnormal.

* Posterior fundus contact lens is a modified Koeppe lens.

* Epidemic kerato conjunctivitis can be spread by tonometry.

* Perimetry is a relatively rough test & purely subjective.

* An accurate assessment of the corneal surface may be made by **Placido's keratoscopic disc.**

* Definite blue coloration of the circumcorneal sclera, is pathological in all except **young children.**

* The corneal endothelium is examined by the **Clinical specular microscope.**

* The most popular applanation tonometer was designed by Goldmann for use with the **Haag-Streit Slit-lamp.**

* **Klein Keratoscopy** is used to study the regularity of the corneal light reflection in the examination of suspected Keratoconus.

* Ultrasonography can detect retinal detachment.

* The **Amsler grid** is useful for detecting and following central scotomas.

* **Strongest** mydriatic (cycloplegic) agent is atropine.

* Sulphonamides are the most commonly incriminated group of drugs in the causation of the Stevens Johnson syndrome.

* 10% phenylephrine drops should not be used in neonates, cardiac patients and patient's receiving antidepressants.

* Topical steroids are contraindicated in superficial viral keratitis, bacterial corneal ulcer and keratomycosis.

* Both glaucoma & cataract are ocular side effects of systemic steroids.

* Intravitreal injection is the most effective route of administration in endophthalmitis.

* On instillation of the medicated drops the permeability of the drug into the eye is mainly determined by the epithelium of cornea.

* Topical treatment of phlyctenular conjunctivitis is by steroid drops.

* Acycloguanosine is the antiviral drug effective against Herpes simplex stromal infection.

* The most effective antiviral drug against Herpes simplex and zoster virus is Ganciclovir.

* Zinc sulphate eye drops is effective in the treatment of angular conjunctivitis.

* Pilocarpine, 1% should be instilled at the end of the examination in all eyes that have been dilated with phenylephrine, (to prevent an attack of acute angle-closure glaucoma, if the AC angle is narrow).

* The condition of spasm of accommodation can be best diagnosed by the use of atropine.

* Tetracycline eye ointment is the drug of choice for control of mass infection of trachoma and in trachoma control programme.

* Accommodation is not involved by epinephrine.

* Retrobulbar injections of steroids in the inflammatory conditions of posterior segment of the eye are ineffective.

* All the antibiotics are inactivated by the heavy metals (lotions containing zinc or mercury should not be prescribed along with them).

* Sulphonamides are indicated in intra-ocular infections and penicillin is most generally useful in extra-ocular infections.

* Carbolic acid cauterisation causes more pain than Tincture Iodine cauterisation.

* Most drugs which dilate the pupil also paralyse the accommodation.

* Miosis may be induced by histamine.

* Sulfonamides are effective against chlamydial group of organisms.

* Ointments cause blurring of the vision.

* Initial drug of choice for most mycotic corneal ulcers is **Natamycin.**

* The adverse ocular effect of vitamin D is band shaped keratopathy.

* Mydriatics and cycloplegic drugs work more effectively on blue eyes than on brown eyes.

* Ointments have greater therapeutic effectiveness than solutions.

* Unsupervised self-administration of local anaesthetics is dangerous.

* Prolonged use of corticosteroids is sometimes complicated by fungal infection.

* **Hutchinson's Freckle**—(lentigo maligna)—Epithelial melanosis—superficially spreads in elderly individuals.

* **Butcher's conjunctivitis**—Fluid from a dead Ascaris lumbricoides worm may get into eye and produce painful & severe conjunctivitis.

* **Pseudomembranes**—Coagulated, exudate adherent to the inflammed conjunctival epithelium seen in —
  * Severe adenoviral infection.
  * Ligneous conjunctivitis
  * Gonococcal conjunctivitis
  * Autoimmune conjunctivitis.

* **True membranes**—Inflammatory exudate permeates the superficial layers of conjunctival epithelium. Seen in :
  * Diphtheria
  * β-haemolytic streptococci

* Any discharge even a watery secretion from a baby's eyes during the 1st week of neonatal period should be viewed with suspicion since tears are not secreted of this early date.

* **Leber cells**—Trachoma follicle contains large multinucleated cells and tend to show necrosis, scarring.

* **Giemsa stain** is the most common stain used when conjunctival scrapings are taken for evaluation.

* The eyes should not be bandaged in Acute catarrhal or mucopurulent conjunctivitis.

* Conjunctiva is rich in lymphatics.

* Hyperemia is the **most conspicuous clinical sign** of acute conjunctivitis.

* Sjogren's syndrome should be considered in any patient with dry eye.

* Itching of the eye is an important feature of allergic conjunctivitis (itching is not seen in bacterial or viral conjunctivitis)

* The best instruments for optic nerve evaluation and determination of cup/disc ratio are the direct ophthalmoscope or the 90D volk lens (indirect ophthalmoscope should not be used).

* The bacterial content of the conjunctival sac is increased by bandaging (due to increase temperature of sac and absence of lid movements).

* **N. catarrhalis** is rarely found in acute conjunctivitis, but more often in chronic and postoperative forms.

* Every case of membranous conjunctivitis should be treated as diphtherial unless good negative evidence is afforded by films and cultures.

* Unilateral chronic conjunctivitis should suggest the presence of a foreign body retained in the fornix, or inflammation of the lacrimal sac.

* Haemorrhagic conjunctivitis is due to the picornavirus.

* Cornybacterium xerosis is frequently present in the normal conjunctival sac.

* **Arlt's line** is present in Trachoma.

* **'Sun-grain' and 'sago-grain' follicles** are characteristic of trachoma.
* Pannus formation is seen in the stage II of trachoma.
* Intraepithelial bullae formation occurs in pemphigus.
* Staphylococci can cause blepharitis, keratitis and conjunctivitis.
* Preauricular lymphadenopathy is a feature of viral & chlamydial conjunctivitis but is seldom present in bacterial conjunctivitis.
* Epidemic keratoconjunctivitis is the only serious eye disease known to be transmissible by tonometry.
* Limbal papillae are characteristic of vernal keratoconjunctivitis, rare in atopic keratoconjunctivitis.
* Phlyctenules are localized manifestations of microbial allergy.
* Both vernal keratoconjunctivitis and limbic keratoconjunctivitis may be associated with keratoconus.
* Difficulty in keeping the eyes open is a common symptom of simple chronic conjunctivitis.
* Trachoma pannus requires no special treatment for it quietness with the recession of the conjunctival activity.
* Conjunctival ulceration should always suggest either the presence of an embedded foreign body or a tuberculous or syphilitic lesion.
* Patient with vernal keratoconjunctivitis (spring catarrh) have an increased incidence of keratoconus.
* If there is chronic conjunctivitis unilateral one should suspect retained foreign body in the fornix or trichiasis or chronic dacryocystitis.
* Basophilic response is present in vernal conjunctivitis.
* Vision in pterygium is impaired with the encroachment of pupillary area and fibrosis in pterygium resulting in astigmatism.
* The **most binding** sequelae of trachoma is entropion with trichiasis.
* Vernal conjunctivitis flares up in summer season.
* Rarely deficiency of the vitamin B_6 is associated with angular conjunctivitis.
* Spring catarrh secretions contain eosinophils.

* Multinuclear giant cells are found in trachoma.
* All signs of trachoma are more severe in the upper than lower conjunctiva.
* The most common conspicious clinical sign of acute conjunctivitis is **Hyperemia.**
* A bilateral transmissible disease of children characterised by numerous follicles in the upper and lower tarsal conjunctiva which is self-limiting is called **Chronic follicular conjunctivitis (orphan's conjunctivitis, Axenfeld's conjunctivitis).**
* A grossly visible preauricular node is an important sign of **Parinaud's Oculoglandular syndrome.**
* Minute hard yellow spots in the palpebral conjunctiva due to accumulation of epithelial cells and inspissated mucus in depression called Henle's gland is called **Concretion ("Lithiasis").**
* **Cornea plana**—Flattening of the anterior contour of cornea, marked astigmatism occurs.
* **Keratoglobus**—Bilateral enlargement of cornea with globular shape and causes myopic & astigmatic refractive errors.
* **Nebula**—thin corneal scar results in slight opacity.
* **Hudson-Stahli lines**—Brown pigmented line in the cornea caused by the deposit of intracytoplasmic iron due to trauma (alkali burns).
* **Krukenberg's spindle**—Accumulation of vertical spindle shaped pigment on the back of corneal endothelium due to breakdown of iris pigment and is seen in pigmentary glaucoma, trauma, iritis & diabetes.
* **Thygeson's superficial punctate keratitis**—Coarse punctate epithelial keratitis with exacerbations & remissions, with foreign body sensation, photophobia and tearing bilaterally and responds to typical steroids.
* **Terrien's marginal degeneration**—Noninflammatory thinning of the margins of cornea.
* **Wessley type of immune ring**—Seen in keratitis disciform is with slit lamp examination.

* **Reis-Buckler's corneal dystrophy**—AD, arises in Bowman's membrane, irregular dense grey subepithelial opacities arranged in **fish-net pattern.**

* **Meesmann's corneal dystrophy**—Meesmann's corneal dystrophy onset in infancy, clear epithelial microcysts, vision unaffected, symptomatic treatment.

* **Schnyder's crystalline dystrophy**—AD, round ring-shaped central corneal opacity consisting of cholesterol crystals.

* **Commonest** form of suppurative keratitis—> Corneal ulcer (Saucer shaped usually).

* Purulent iridocyclitis/Panophthalmitis may be set up in a perforated corneal ulcer, especially in gonococcal ophthalmia and Hypopyon ulcer.

* Steroids should be discontinued since they may retard epithelialization and inhibit repair by fibrosis (once the inflammation ceases).

* **Cauterisation** of the progressive corneal ulcer may be performed with pure carbolic acid or trichloroacetic Acid (10-20%).

* **Hypopyon ulcer—causative organism**
  * Pneumococcus
  * E. coli
  * Moraxella
  * Streptococci
  * Ps. Pyocyanea
  * B. aerogenes
  * B. subtilis

* Antiviral drugs are not advised, as they may induce scarring beneath the lesions in **Thygeson's** superficial punctate keratitis.

* Silver nitrate cautery sticks should not be used for local application in superior limbic kerato conjunctivitis (as severe conjunctival burn and necrosis can occur).

* The most important factor in maintaining corneal transparency is the ability of the cornea to keep itself relatively dehydrated.

* Chromatic aberration is seen in patients with corneal edema.

* The **most effective** treatment for the ocular manifestations of acne rosacea is systemic tetracycline.

* Stratified squamous epithelium covers the cornea.

* Pseudocornea has only two layers i.e. connective tissue layers with epithelium.

* Poor antigenecity of the corneal stroma is due to avascularity, sparse cell count had separation of cells by ground substance.

* **Keratocele** refers to herniation of Descemet's membrane.

* Stromal herpes keratitis and iritis are best treated with Acycloguanosine.

* The most effective antifungal agent in candida infection is Tinactin (Nystatin).

* Timolol should not be used in the treatment of corneal ulcer.

* **Ulcus serpens** is caused by pneumococcus.

* Hypopyon ulcer is most often seen with pneumococcus.

* In an established case of keratoconus the best treatment is penetrating keratoplasty.

* Permanent scarring occur if there is damage to Bowman's membrane.

* The safe and the best treatment of exposure keratitis is Tarsorrhaphy till the lagophthalmos recovers.

* Lamellar keratoplasty is the treatment of choice for Mooren's ulcer.

* Cornea guttata is seen in the endothelial dystrophy of Fuchs.

* Corneal dystrophy shows **'fish net pattern'** of corneal opacities.

* Longstanding corneal odema is best treated with whole thickness corneal graft.

* Intraocular pressure is elevated in buphthalmos but normal in megalocornea.

* **Mooren's ulcer** never perforates the cornea.

* Corneal thickness is measured by pachometer and smoothness or irregularities of corneal surface are detected by Placido's disc.

* The most accepted treatment of impending corneal perforation is therapeutic keratoplasty.

* The corneal epithelium restricts the passage of fluid because of the presence of Desmosomes.

* Central nebula produces greatest visual impairment.

* Arcus juvenilis occurs in Hypercholesterolaemia.
* Ocular complications are usually associated with the involvement of Nasocilliary nerve.
* Dystrophy occurring in patient who have suffered from previous corneal disease is Salzman's nodular dystrophy.
* Steroids are indicated topically indisciform keratitis.
* Pseudo-hypopyon is found in tuberculous iritis.
* Dendritic corneal ulcers are characteristic of Herpes simplex keratitis.
* Keratitis disciformis is due to antigen reaction in the stroma.
* In keratoconus the cone is situated just below the centre of the cornea.
* The reservoir of infection in herpes zoster ophthalmicus is Gasserian ganglion.
* **Reis-Buckler corneal dystrophy** commonly shows recurrent corneal erosions.
* Keratoconus does not cause fold in Descemet's membrane.
* In Keratoconus the cone is situated just below the centre of the cornea.
* Systemic steroids are recommended in herpes zoster ophthalmicus when associated with progressive proptosis, total 3rd nerve palsy and optic neuritis.
* Congenital syphilis shows **'star map' keratic precipitates.**
* The nerve which is rarely involved in herpes zoster ophthalmicus is infra-orbital nerve.
* Best treatment of keratocele or descemetocele is rest and pressure bandage.
* KP's are a feature of keratomalacia.
* Intraocular tension is raised in corneal ulcer.
* Epithelial abrasion of cornea results in nebula grade opacity.
* The most characteristic lesion due to Herpes simplex virus infection is **Dendritic ulcer.**
* When a phlyctena migrates from the limbus towards the centre of the cornea and carries a leash of blood vessels with it from the limbus, it is known as **Fascicular ulcer.**

* Corneal degeneration due to exposure to ultraviolet light, characterised by fine subepithelial yellow droplets in peripheral cornea which becomes central with blurred vision is known as **Climatic droplet keratopathy (Pearl divers keratopathy, spheroid degeneration of the cornea).**

* Fungi can penetrate an intact Descemet's membrane.

* **Bergmeister's papilla**—Is a remnant of the hyaloid vascular system.

* **Mittendorf dot**—Is a remnant of the hyaloid vascular system.

* **Foster Fuch's Fleck**—Circular claret coloured or Black spot at the Fovea suddenly formed due to choroidal thrombosis. (Is seen in pathological myopia at the macula).

* **Junius-Kuhnt's disease**—Disciform degeneration of Macula.

* **Hilding syndrome**—Destructive iridocyclitis with multiple joint dislocation.

* **Lewis syndrome**—Tuberoserpiginous syphilis of Lewis.

* **Parry-Romberg syndrome**—Progressive facial hemiatrophy.

* **Scleral thinning** is seen in :
    * Uveitis
    * Scleritis
    * Tuberculoma

* **Conglomerate Tubercle**—> The presence of satellites, usual absence of visible vein upon the surface of the nodules, The age of the patient and presence of iritis distinguish it from a malignant melanoma.

* **Koeppee's Nodules**—> Minute transparent Nodules appear on the surface of the iris at pupillary border—exudative type of Tuberculous iritis.

* Subconjunctival injections of steroids are contraindicated in scleritis (because of fear of rupture of the globe).

* The agent contraindicated in the treatment of toxoplasmosis with pyremethamine is Folic acid.

* Contraindications to surgical treatment of iridocyclitis include ↑ IOP, KP and exudative choroiditis.

* Patient with aniridia have a higher prevalence of Wilm's tumor.

* Choroid is lined by membrane of Bruch.

* The diseases of sclera are chronic because of relative avascularity of sclera.

* Episcleral vessels are dilated in Glaucoma, cortico-venous fistula and Endocrine exophthalmos.

* Gonorrhoeal iritis is characterised by a peculiar gelatinous, greenish grey coloured exudates in AC.

* Syphilitic iritis manifests itself as either simple plastic iritis or Gummatous iritis.

* An active lesion of choroiditis gives rise to positive scotoma.

* Malignant melanoma of the uvea does not cause metastasis.

* Aqueous flare seen in AC is due to the out pouring of leucocytes in the AC & minute flakes of coagulated proteins.

* Sarcoidosis & Behcet's syndrome show ↑ IgA levels.

* KP in iridocyclitis are seen on the back of endothelial cells over the triangular area of the lower part of the cornea.

* Disciform lesions at the macula are seen in exudative age related macular disease and presumed ocular histoplasma syndrome.

* When choroiditis occurring close to the disc is known as Juxtapapillary choroiditis.

* The strength attachment of the vitreous body is to the **Vitreous base.**

* Vitreous never regenerates.

* The **earlier sign** of an iritis is endothelial bedwing of the cornea.

* **'Episcleritis periodica fugax'** is so named because the attacks are fleeting and frequently repeated.

* The strongest attachment of the vitreous humour is to the ora serrata.

* Bilateral, punched out, heavily pigmented retinochoroidal scars in the macular region are seen in toxoplasmosis.

* Persistent pupillary membrane is a remnant of anterior vascular sheath of the lens.

* 50% of cases of scleritis is associated with connective tissue disease.

* The teritary vitreous corresponds to the Zonule of Zinn.
* The best way of diagnosing subretinal neovascular membrane is by Florescein angiography.
* The lesion in the choroid are restricted to isolated areas because of segmental blood supply to choroid.
* The conditions mimicking vitreous detachment are normal vitreous, membrane formation in the vitreous and Cloquet's canal.
* Glaucoma in essential iris atrophy is caused by the down-growth of an endothelial membrane over the tissue at the angle of AC.
* Small pupil in iridocyclitis is due to leased acting as irritant and causing constrictor pupillae to contract.
* Colloid bodies or drusen are the excrescences of Bruch's membrane and are said to be secreted from pigment epithelial cells.
* Uveitis with iris atrophy is seen in Herpes zoster.
* Ankylosing spondylosis is commonly associated with uveitis.
* Inflammation of choroid always involves the retina because of dependence of outer half of the retina for its blood supply of choroid.
* Iridocyclitis may give rise to complicated cataract.
* A virulent form of diffuse annular scleritis, usually bilateral and associated with gelatinous swelling of the episcleral tissue is known as **Brawny scleritis.**
* Scleral disease characterised by thinning and melting of the scleral tissue, leading to areas of dehiscence without any history or clinical evidence of inflammation of the sclera usually associated with rheumatoid conditions is termed as **Necrotising scleromalacia (scleromalacia perforans).**
* The glass ball inserted into the sclera following evisceration is known as **Artificial Vitreous (MULES' operation).**
* The presence of glittering crystals in liquified vitreous often consisting of cholesterol and due to longlasting degenerative changes is called **Synchisis scintillans.**
* The frequent cause of anterior uveitis associated with a marked preponderance in males is **Marie Strumpell ankylosing spondylitis.**

* Early and constant pupillary dilatation reduces the incidence of posterior synechia.
* Vitreous loss is an iatrogenic complication.
* The lens is incapable of becoming inflammed due to the capsule.
* Needling of lamellar cataract—done at 3 years of age.

Types of pupillary reflex :

* Cataracta nigra	—	Black
* Cataracta brunescens	—	Brownish
* Immature senile cataract	—	Greyish white
* Mature senile cataract	—	Pearly white
* Hypermature Morgagnian cataract	—	Milky white
* Aphakia	—	Jet white
* Calcium deposition	—	Chalky white
* Glaucoma	—	Sea green

Purkinje Sanson images :

(Seen in darken room with candle light or pen torch)

* 1st image	—	Anterior surface of cornea
* 2nd image	—	Posterior surface of cornea
* 3rd image	—	Anterior lens surface
* 4th image	—	Posterior lens surface

Interpretation of Purkinje Sanson image :

* 1st and 4th image	—	Clearly visible
* 2nd and 4th image darkrom	—	Seen in bright light in
* If 4th image is absent	—	Lens is opaque
* If 4th image is present	—	Lens is clear
* If 3rd and 4th images	—	Aphakia (absence of lens)

* 1st, 2nd and 3rd images move with the movement of light. (Convex surfaces).
* **'Cataract nigra lens' (Black cataract):** Deposition of melanin pigment over the senile nucleus sclerotic lens gives black colour.

* Lenticular rosette formation is usually associated with concussion cataract.

* The best method to decide about the immaturity and maturity of senile cataract is distant direct ophthalmoscopy.

* The safe and best treatment of posterior capsule thickening is non-invasive laser capsulotomy and the type of laser employed includes YAG laser.

* Concussion cataract is due to rupture of lens capsule.

* Suggested treatment for secondary glaucoma following intumescent cataract is lens extraction.

* Rosette shaped cataract is usually seen in posterior cortex.

* **Elschnig's pearls** (balloon like cells seen in after cataract) are derived from subcapsular epithelial cells of the iris.

* The **safest** method of an intracapsular extraction employed in an intumescent cataract is cryoprobe.

* The posterior polar cataract may diminish the vision considerably because it is close to the nodal point of eye.

* Cupliform or posterior cortical cataract never matures.

* Malignant glaucoma is produced after surgery.

* The indication of early surgery in congenital cataract is development of nystagmus and squint.

* Steroid induced cataract shows posterior subcapsular opacity.

* **Water cleft** is present in immature cortical cataract.

* Vitreous loss during cataract extraction can be anticipated when the patient is young who has short and thick neck with narrowed palpebral fissure.

* Cataract associated with galactosaemia is deep cortical.

* Nuclear sclerosis causes change in the refractive state of the eye towards myopia.

* Lens striae make their appearance in the lower and nasal quadrant.

* Total lenticular opacity in a child is best treated by aspiration.

* If the vision of the patient is worse in bright light and better in semidark room the type of opacity in the lens is central.

* The presence of glutathione and ascorbic acid in the lens may serve as agents for oxygen transfer.

* The clinical evidence of irradiation cataract is apparent in the cortex near the posterior pole after a period of **1 to 2 years.**

* Coloboma of the lens which is usually seen in the inferior margin is due to defective development of part of the suspensory ligament.

* The anterior chamber is deep in Aphakia.

* Senile cataracts in diabetics develop at an early age.

* Blue dot cataract causes visual disturbance.

* Linear opacities like spokes of a wheel are seen in zonular cataracts.

* Discission operation may require repetition.

* The main cause of development of cataract following renal transplantation is due to **use of immunosuppressive drugs.**

* The intrauterine infection of a protozoan causing cataract is **Toxoplasmosis.**

* The surgical technique for cataract extraction using a probe that vibrates at ultrasonic frequency and emulsifies the lens nucleus is **Phacoemulsification.**

* The eponymous name for traumatic cataract caused by the imprint of the iris pigment on the anterior surface of the lens is **Vossius' cataract or ring.**

* The type of laser used for posterior capsulotomy is **Nd; YAG (neodymium; yitrium aluminium garnet) laser.**

* Iridodonesis is a common sign of lens dislocation.

* Patient with opacity/dislocation of lens will complain of blurred vision without pain.

* Traumatic glaucoma cases are commonly caused by angle recession.

* The congenital anomaly most commonly associated with Buphthalmos is facial haemangiomas.

* **Barkan's membrane**—Covers the trabecular meshwork in primary infantile glaucoma.

* **Prosner-Schlossman syndrome**—Glaucomatocyclitic crisis.

* **Sampaolesi's line syndrome**—Heavy pigment deposition in the chamber angle and in a line above Schwalbe's line (Exfoliation glaucoma).
* Pilocarpine and carbachol are contraindicated in inflammatory glaucoma, malignant glaucoma or known allergy.
* Phenylephrine should not be used in closed-angle glaucoma.
* Timolol eye drops are contraindicated in bronchial asthma and patients of bradycardia and heart blocks.
* Epinephrine is **contraindicated** in narrow angle glaucoma or known allergy.
* Anticholinesterase agents (Echothiopate iodide and Demecarium bromide) are contraindicated in uveitis and narrow angle glaucoma.
* Carbonic anhydrase inhibitors (acetazolamide etc.) are contraindicated in patient with significant respiratory disease, known allergy.
* Haemorrhage glaucoma is due to neovascularization of angle.
* Removal of lens is the treatment for malignant glaucoma.
* The rise of IOP is due to difficulty in its exit from AC.
* The most preferred site for filtering operation is superior nasal quadrant.
* Argon laser trabeculoplasty is only adjuvant to glaucoma therapy.
* Phacolytic type of lens protein glaucoma is due to phagocytes laden with lens protein which block the trabeculum.
* As per the diurnal variation of IOP, it is least at 8.00 a.m.
* Visual acuity and visual field loss are reversible upto stage of constant instability.
* The most useful gonioscopic sign in angle recession glaucoma is greater space between the iris root and the scleral spur.
* The dark room prone test is the provocative test for primary narrow angle glaucoma.
* **Krukenberg's spindle** of pigment is seen on the endothelium of the cornea.
* Enucleation operation is best suited for absolute glaucoma treatment.

* **Ocular hypertension** is a term applied to patient having chronic elevation of IOP without field defects.

* In acute congestive glaucoma the pupil is large, oval and long axis vertical.

* 35% of patients of pigment dispersion syndrome develop pigmentary glaucoma.

* **Glaucoma capsulare** follows exfoliation of the superficial layers of the lens capsule.

* Peripheral iridectomy should be performed in the prodromal stage of glaucoma.

* Lens extraction is the correct surgical procedure in secondary glaucoma following hypermature Morgagnian cortical cataract.

* The classical symptom of prodromal stage of angle closure glaucoma is Halos and which are due to corneal oedema

* In patient of open angle glaucoma the cup/disc ratio ↑ with time.

* Plateau iris is a variant of angle closure.

* Miotics are not useful in — Buphthalmos, Aphakic glacuoma, Glaucomatocyclitic crisis, Glaucoma inversus and in epidemic dropsy glaucoma.

* **Mackay Marg tonometer** is suitable to record tension in the presence of corneal oedema.

* Delayed dark adaptation and frequent changes of near vision glasses are the symptoms of open angle glaucoma.

* If the normal outflow through canal of schlemm is blocked the alternate route is through uveoscleral outflow.

* Infantile glaucoma is due to anterior insertion of iris than usual, non-separation of the iris from the cornea and failure in the development of structures in angle of AC.

* Direct visualization of the angle of AC is possible with Koeppe lens.

* A cycloplegic drug in a patient with shallow AC is dangerous because it can precipitate an attack of narrow angle glaucoma.

* Cornea, iris and retinal structures of the eye are enlarged in Buphthalmos (but lens is not enlarged).

* Secondary glaucoma after perforation of the cornea is due to blockade of the drainage angle by anterior synechiae.

* In trabeculectomy the aqueous humour is drained by transcleral route to subconjunetival space and two open ends of the canal of schlemm.

* Hypermetropic eyes are vulnerable to have attack of narrow angle glaucoma.

* The most significant test in low tension glaucoma is Tonography.

* Painful eye of absolute glaucoma can be treated by cyclodialysis, cyclodiathermy and cycloanaemization.

* In an acute congestive glaucoma the choice of surgery between peripheral iridectomy and filtering operation is decided by Gonioscopic examination.

* Tonometry is an important test in the diagnosis of glaucoma.

* Dilation of the pupil should be avoided if anterior chamber is shallow.

* The earliest and most constant symptom in infantile glaucoma is **Epiphora.**

* Glaucoma associated with a hypermature cataract, caused by blockage of the trabecular meshwork by phagocytes containing lens matter is termed as **Phacolytic glaucoma.**

* An elevated intraocular pressure without evidence of anatomic or functional damage to the eye denotes **Ocular hypertension.**

* A type of trauma induced unilateral secondary glaucoma following a contussion injury associated with deep anterior chamber is **Angle recession glaucoma.**

* Surgery upon an eye with markedly increased intraocular pressure and a closed angle can lead to **Ciliary block glaucoma (Malignant glaucoma).**

* Diurnal pressure curves disclose the real diagnosis in low pressure glaucoma.

* Cataract surgery and open angle glaucoma surgery may be done simultaneously.

* **Septic Retinitis of Roth :**
  * Typically in Bacterial endocarditis and some time in purulent septicaemia—posterior part of the fundus is affected.
  * Numerous recurrent haemorrhages of embolic origin, some of them with white centres as in anaemias.
  * Characteristic feature—>*Roth's spots* (round/oval white spots)—>(Cytoid bodies).
  * Some oedema and papilloedema may occur.
  * The disease is frequently fatal and vision is seriously impaired.
* 'Sea-fan' neovascularisation is most commonly seen in sickle-cell haemoglobin C disease and sickle thalassemia.
* In branch retinal vein occlusion (BRVO), the superotemporal quadrant of the retina is most commonly affected (33%).
* There is a high incidence of anterior segment neovascularisation with CRVO which results in severe glaucoma.
* **Paving stone or cobblestone degeneration** lesions are found in the inferior temporal quadrants (in three quarter of cases).
* Exudative cells in the overlying vitreous are common in toxoplasmosis.
* Ocular complications are seen in sickle cell C disease and sickle cell thalassemia.
* Coat's disease is the most severe form of retinal telangiectasia.
* Rods are primarily affected in retinitis pigmentosa.
* The accepted treatment of clinically significant macular oedema of diabetes is laser photocoagulation.
* The thickest area of the sensory retina is located in the proximity of the optic disc.
* Lattice degeneration occurs in the supero-temporal quadrant.
* The most effective treatment in CRA occlusion is ocular massage.
* Blurring of the optic disc margin occurs in papillitis.
* Hand exudates are due to phagocytosis of degenerated retinal tissue by macrophages which undergo hyaline degeneration.
* Henle's fibre layer is the synaptic interconnection of the photoreceptors with the bipolar cells occurring in the outer plexiform layer.

* SLE enhances the toxic effect of chloroquine on retina.
* **Cattle-truck appearance** is seen in incomplete obstruction of CRA.
* Visual evoked response (VER) indicates the state of the Foveal region.
* Cystoid macular oedema occurs because of breakdown of inner retinal barrier.
* The neuron of the second order in the retina is ganglion cells.
* Nerve fibres in the nerve layer of the retina are non-medullated.
* Indirect ophthalmoscopy is most useful in diagnosis of retinal holes.
* Cytomegaloviral retinitis is seen in patient who are receiving immunosuppressive agents and suffering from HIV infection.
* The most characteristic finding of an exudative retinal detachment is shifting subretinal fluid.
* Retinal haemorrhages with characteristic white centres are called as **Roth's spots.**
* In fluorescein angiography the dye is injected into the antecubital vein.
* In toxaemia of pregnancy the termination of pregnancy should be advised with the advent of cotton wool spots.
* The capillaries of the CRV are found in the inner nuclear layer and nerve fibre layer.
* **Hollenhorst's plaques** are derived from atheromatous plaques.
* The early sign of the background diabetic retinopathy is microaneurysm in the macular area.
* Reversal of diabetic retinopathy is seen in woman with Sheehan's syndrome (due to lack of growth hormone).
* Diabetic patient with HLA-B$_{15}$ are more likely to develop proliferative retinopathy.
* Mother who are antibody positive or who have had one child with congenital toxoplasmosis will not give birth to a child with congenital toxiplasmosis (Because acute toxoplasma infecton occurs only once).

* Choriodermia (retinal degeneration) has an X-linked recessive inheritance, therefore, males are affected and females are carriers.
* The cardinal symptom of macular disease is blurring of central vision.
* Colour vision is not significantly impaired in eyes with early macular disease, in contrast to eyes with early lesions of the optic nerve.
* **Salt and pepper retinopathy** is seen in Leber's amaurosis, congenital rubella and congenital syphilis.
* **Macular star** is due to papilloedema, hypertensive retinopathy and Eale's disease.
* **Beaten bronze atrophy** of the foveal region is seen in Stargardt's disease.
* Findings of sickle cell retinopathy are most prominent in superior temporal retina.
* Leber's miliary aneurysms are found in Coat's disease.
* The rods and cones as well as the outer nuclear layers are not affected in Stargardt's disease.
* The peripheral part of the ocular fundus is best examined by indirect ophthalmoscopy and scleral indentation.
* Normal EOG is seen in **Oguchi's disease.**
* In the detachment of retina it is the pigment layer which separates from neurosensory retina.
* Flame shaped superficial haemorrhage occurs in the nerve fibre layer of the retina.
* Localised narrowing of the retinal arterioles occurs in Hypertensive retinopathy and Toxaemia of pregnancy.
* In a young child related to a family of retinitis pigmentosa the early diagnosis is achieved by ERG (electro-retinogram) and EOG (electro-oculogram).
* Retinal arterial pulsations are seen in aortic regurgitation, dysthyroid exophthalmos and orbital tumours.
* The best method of examining the details of retinal detachment is indirect ophthalmoscopy.

* Retinal white with pressure is seen in retinal holes.
* **'Scrambled egg appearance'** in the foveal region is found in Best's disease.
* The shape of subhyaloid haemorrhage is first round and then quickly become hemispherical.
* Retinitis pigmentosa is an atrophy of the retina.
* Retinal holes are frequently difficult to find.
* Background retinal abnormalities are confined to the retina.
* Diabetic retinopathy is often bilateral.
* The appearance on the retinae of hypertensive subjects under the light of the ophthalmoscope of thickened arteries in which the light reflex becomes brilliantly white is known as **"Silver wire arteries"**.
* A condition of retinal oedema, which consists of rapid, usually temporary loss of visual acuity in aphakic patients commonly after intracapsular extraction is known as **Irvine-Gass syndrome.**
* The distinctive feature of retinal tear is an **Operculum of avulsed tissue.**
* A bilateral retinal disease of premature infants is **Retrolental fibroplasia.**
* The application of light energy in the form of ordinary light ray or laser beam that is absorbed by the blood present in ocular tissues, which causes disruption of the cells with formation of scar tissue is known as **Photocoagulation.**
* The splitting of the retina into two layers, the dehiscence usually being between the receptors and bipolar cells is known as **Retinoschisis.**
* Disease of the retinal vessels is almost invariably associated with disease of the cerebral vessels.
* **Hollenhorst plaque (cholesterol emboli)**—Break off ulcerative atheroma of internal carotid artery and enters retinal circulation (CRA closure).
* **Cowen's sign**—jerky pupillary constriction on a consensual light stimulus (Graves' disease).

* **Romberg's sign**—Unsteadiness of balance when eyes are closed.

* **"Morning glory" syndrome**—Unilateral dysplastic coloboma cup filled with glial tissue and surrounded by pigment ring, spoke-like radiation of vessles, with retinal detachment and poor vision.

* **One and a half syndrome**—Unilateral pontine lesion, affects horizontal gaze centre and medial longitudinal fasciculus, ipsilateral gaze palsy internuclear ophthalmoplegia and only movement is abduction in contralateral eye with ataxic nystagmus (seen in multiple scleosis, basilar artery occlusion and pontine metastasis).

* **In infancy pupil is smaller than at birth.**
  * At age 1—pupil begins to widen.
  * Reaches greatest diameter during adolescence.
  * Again smaller with advancing age.
  * Myopes have larger pupils than hyperopes.
  * Normal diameter — 3 to 4 mm.
  * Mydriatic & cycloplegics work more effectively on blue eyes than on brown eyes.

* **Physiological constriction of pupil :**
  * Light reflex
  * Direct light reflex
  * Consensual light reflex
  * Convergence near reflex
  * Accommodation near reflex

* Papilloedema is hydrostatic non-inflammatory phenomenon. Due to CRV compression as it crosses the subdural and subarachnoid spaces also due to Hypoxia of the tissues at the nerve head.

* The classical sign of chiasmal visual field involvement is bitemporal hemianopia (these defects do not cross the vertical midline).

* **See-saw nystagmus** is usually associated with bitemporal hemianopia and third ventricular tumors.

* **"Pie in the sky"**—Superior right homonymous quadrantic defect is due to a lesion of the most anterior inferior fibres of the optic radiations in the temporal lobe (**Meyer's loop**).

* **"Pie in the floor"**—Complete right inferior homonymous quadrantanopia due to a lesion of the superior fibres of the optic radiations in the left parietal lobe.

* Anterior optic tract lesion produces an incongruous homonymous hemianopia, decreased visual acuity, afferent pupil defect (**Wernicke's hemianopic pupil**) and atrophy of the optic discs with bow-tie atrophy in the contralateral eye.

* Leber's disease affects males predominantly.

* 3 tests to confirm diagnosis of Horner's syndrome are :
  * Cocaine test
  * Paredrine test
  * Dilatation lag

* Visual field defects associated with papilledema are enlarged blind spot and constriction of the peripheral field.

* Hippus (alternating pupillary size) is a **prominent** sign in multiple sclerosis.

* ARP is due to lesion in tectum.

* Field defect in papilledema is by enlargement of blind spot and progressive contraction of the visual field.

* Gold perimetry is the best investigation for optic neuritis.

* Optic nerve carries the axons of neurones of the second order.

* Diagnosis of optic neuritis based on perimetry is clinched by the presence of central scotoma.

* Absence of sustained pupillary constriction is the diagnostic sign of retrobulbar optic neuritis.

* Optic nerve is enclosed within meningeal sheath upto the lamina cribrosa.

* A typical diabetic oculomotor palsy is ischaemic.

* Visual centres are the site of lesion in uraemic amaurosis.

* Tumours of the orbital surface of the frontal lobe causes Foster-Kennedy syndrome.

* Macular sparing occurs in suprageniculate lesions of visual pathways.

* Gaze evoked amaurosis is seen in optic nerve sheath meningioma.

* Optic nerve lesions typically produce negative scotomas whereas macular lesions cause positive scotomas.

* Papilledema is a major ophthalmic and neurologic emergency and patient requires immediate admission to hospital.

* Always suspect the diagnosis of giant cell arteritis in every elderly patient with amaurosis fugax, ischemic optic neuropathy, CRA occlusion and/or suggestive systemic symptomatology.

* A patient with elevated ESR and symptoms of giant cell arteritis should have a temporal artery biopsy.

* **Paredrine test** can separate a third neurone Horner's syndrome from first and second neuron syndromes.

* There is no pharmacologic test that can differentiate a first and second neuron Horner's syndrome (These must be identified clinically by the associated brainstem (**first neuron**) or spinal cord and lung apex (**second neuron**) symptoms and signs.

* A single lesion situated at the junction of nerve and chiasma can produce visual field defects in both eyes.

* Papilledema is nearly always bilateral.

* ARP results in the lesions between the decussation and the constrictor centre in the mid brain.

* Marcus Gunn pupil is an indication of optic nerve lesions.

* Lack of sustained constriction of pupil on exposure to bright light is a feature of optic neuritis.

* Optic nerve fibres do not regenerate after section because myelin sheathes are separated by glial tissue and a neurilemma is absent.

* Oculomotor nerve nucleus is located at the level of the superior colliculus whereas Trochlear nerve nucleus is located at the level of inferior colliculus.

* **'String of beads'** sign and retinal angiography is seen in amaurosis fugax.

* Anterior ischaemic optic neuropathy causes altitudinal field defects.

* Unilateral papilledema is seen in cavernous sinus thrombosis.

* Contracaecal scotoma particularly to red objects is seen in Tobacco amblyopia which is due to the degeneration of ganglion cells.

* **Riddoch's phenomenon** is classically seen in lesions of occipital lobe.

* **Scinillating scotomata** and **fortification spectra** can be seen in migraine.

* Profound unilateral loss of vision at the very outset of the disease occurs in papillitis.

* The blurring of margins of the optic disc in papilledema first starts at upper and the lower margins.

* Monocular diplopia with homonymous hemianopia is due to a lesion in the calcarine cortex.

* Drusen of the optic disc is due to impaired axoplasmic transport.

* The cranial nerve showing the longest intracranial course is trochlear nerve which is a pure motor nerve.

* Vitreous opacities are seen in papilledema.

* Smooth enlargement of the optic foramen is seen radiologically in optic nerve glioma.

* Spiral field defects continually contracting are seen in hysterical amblyopia.

* Rapid deterioration of vision with a normal appearing fundus is seen in acute retrobulbar neuritis.

* Persistent neuralgia may be a late manifestation of Herpes zoster.

* Vestibular nystagmus is always of the jerky type.

* Spasm of the near reflex is usually caused by hysteria.

* A rare demyelinating disease of central nervous system characterised by bilateral optic neuritis and paraplegia is known as **Neuromyelitis optica (Devic's disease)**.

* The only symptom of optic nerve atrophy is **loss of vision.**

* The syndrome characterised by paralysis of conjugate upward deviation of the eyes, due to a lesion in the midbrain at the level of the anterior corpora quadrigemia is termed as **Perinaud's syndrome or ophthalmoplegia (pretectal syndrome).**

* Gaze nystagmus is suggestive of lesion of the **Posterior cranial fossa.**

* This rare familial condition consisting of unilateral ptosis at rest followed by a rapid exaggerated elevation of the lid when the mandible is depressed or deviated to opposite side is called **Marcus Gunn phenomenon (Jaw winking syndrome).**

* Disease characterised by involvement of all three extraocular nerves with slowly progressive inability to move the eye, severe early ptosis, normal pupillary reactions and accommodation when associated with pigmentary degeneration of retina, deafness, cardiac conduction defects and neuropathy, it is called **ophthalmoplegia plus or Kearns-Sayre syndrome.**

* Abducens palsy is the most common in Basal meningitis.

* Pappilledema may persist for a long time without permanently affecting vision.

* **Orthophoria**—The eyes remain under dissociation, or in the fusion-free position.

* **Anaphoria** is when both eyes deviate upward.

* **Cataphoria** is when both eyes deviate upward.

* **Cyclophoria**—A deviation of the vertical axis of one or both eyes so that they lose their parallelism with the median plane of the head.

* **Plus cyclophoria**—A tendency of the upper end of the vertical corneal meridian to lean outward, i.e, towards the temples (extorsion).

* **Minus cyclophoria**—A tendency of the upper end of the vertical corneal meridian to lean nose ward (intorsion).

* Esotropia is the most common type of misalignment of the eyes.

* Accommodative esotropia usually starts between the ages of 1 and 3 years.

* The cardinal positions of gaze are six in number.

* Latent nystagmus is seen when either eye is covered.

* Oculo-cardiac reflex can get stimulated after squint surgery, retinal detachment surgery and enucleation.

* The longest extrinsic ocular muscle is the superior oblique.

* The activity of fixation reflex can be demonstrated by optokinetic nystagmus.

* **Post-operative complications following squint surgery include :**
  * Suture abscess
  * Orbital cellulitis
  * Conjunctival cyst
  * Granuloma
* **Down beating vertical nystagmus** is seen with posterior tumor.
* The muscle originated from the attachment to the dural sheath of the optic nerve are superior rectus and medial rectus.
* Squint with restricted ocular motility is caused by strabismus fixus, Duane's retraction syndrome and Browns superior oblique sheath syndrome.
* The greatest asthenopic symptoms are caused by cyclophoria.
* Recession of an extraocular muscle is a muscle weakening operation.
* Cyclophoria produces maximal discomfort and it is the rarest type.
* Synoptophore test is especially recommended for detection of stereopsis
* **Spasmus nutans** resolve spontaneously.
* Negative after images are employed in a test for strabismus to determine the direction of fixation.
* Accommodative esotropia is due to a refractive error of hyperopia (far sightedness).
* Hess screen testing is useful in paralytic squint.
* Labyrinthine nystagmus occurs in the disease of internal ear.
* In concommitant squint the afferent pathways are abnormal.
* **See-saw nystagmus of Maddox** is the pathognomonic of parachiasmal disease.
* The point falling on the horopter is seen by the corresponding points.
* A unilateral lesion of posterior longitudinal bundle leads to inner-nuclear ophthalmoplegia.
* The measuring unit of convergence is **Metre angle.**

* Ocular muscles are never affected in polymyositis.
* Surgery is usually unnecessary in fully accommodative esotropia.
* All the intraocular muscles are supplied by 3rd cranial nerve except, **dilator pupillae.**
* In paralytic squint the secondary deviation is more than primary deviation because of overaction of the contralateral synergist.
* **Bielchowsky phenomenon** is characterised by downward deviation of the covered eye in dissociated hyperdeviation.
* **Haidinger's brushes** can be used for detection of eccentric fixation.
* An accurate assessment of movement of each eye can be obtained by talking the field of fixation with **Lister perimeter.**
* In paralytic squint the head is turned in the direction of action of the paralysed muscle due to an attempt to lessen the diplopia.
* Strabismic amblyopia is treated by occulsion of good eye.
* The angle of the strabismus can be measured by amblyoscope, Lister's perimeter and prism bar cover test.
* The phenomenon of approximating the visuoscope target directly against the fovea and immediately there after against the paramacular area following eye movement is known as eccentric viewing.
* The feature of superior oblique sheath syndrome is marked defect of elevation in adduction.
* False orientation is a necessary accompaniment of binocular diplopia.
* Concommitant squint may be constant and periodic.
* The earlier the onset of strabismus, the worse the prognosis for fusion.
* Paralytic strabismus is uncommon in childhood.
* Strabismus surgery is empirical.
* A negative angle kappa gives false impression of esotropia.
* **Hering's law of equal innervation** states that during any conjugate eye movement, equal and simultaneous innervation flows to the yoke muscle.

* The eponymous name for superior oblique tendon sheath syndrome is **Brown's syndrome.**

* **Unilateral strabismus** is the term which sometimes applied to tilting of the head to compensate for defective vertical movements of one eye.

* **Hirschberg's test** objectively estimates the angle of a heterotropia.

* Non-refractive accommodative esotropia is associated with a AC/A ratio.

* Lancaster's red-green test is similar to the Hess test.

* The amount of synblepharon is very extensive in ankyloblepharon, operation may be contraindicated.

* In complete paralysis of the third nerve resulted ptosis, operation is usually contraindicated on account of the abduction of the eye. (if the lid is raised in these cases the diplopia becomes manifest).

* Irrigation & probing should not be carried out in acute dacryocystitis.

* Blindness following blepharoplasty, is nearly always due to orbital haemorrhage.

* The regurgitation test may be false negative in chronic dacryocystitis with internal fistula.

* **Fasanella-Servat operation** for ptosis is carried out in cases with mild ptosis and levator action of more than **8 mm.**

* The most frequent sign of transference of the symptoms to the opposite side in cavernous sinus thrombosis is paralysis of the opposite lateral rectus.

* The optic foramen is an opening in lesser wing of the sphenoid bone.

* The peculiarities of the lids are loosely attached, extremely thin and hairless.

* Blepharophimosis is present in Down's syndrome, Microphthalmos, Edward's syndrome and Waardenburg's syndrome.

* The tumour which spreads from the intracranial space to the orbit is sphenoidal meningioma.

* The nerve supplying the outer part of the eyelid and conjunctiva is maxillary nerve.
* While incising and curetting a chalazion pointing towards conjunctiva, the incision, should be at right angle to the long axis of tarsal plate.
* Acute ethmoiditis in a child aged three years presents with painful proptosis, periorbital swelling, fever and rhinorrhoea.
* Glands of Krause secrete sweat.
* The **earliest** clinical feature of orbital extension of the basal cell carcinoma of the eyelid is diplopia.
* Distichiasis is a developmental condition.
* The **narrowest** part of the nasolacrimal duct is upper end.
* Ptosis associated with lower lid of the affected side at a higher level than the lower lid of the normal side is seen in Horner's syndrome.
* Orbital mucormycosis occurs most often in patient with **diabetic ketosis.**
* If the eye ball is congenitally absent the condition is called **as congenital anophthalmos.**
* Both bilateral frontalis sling and levator resection are effective in synkinetic ptosis.
* III burns of eyelids should be treated by split skin grafts immediately.
* In dacryocystorhinostomy the communication of the sac is established with middle meatus.
* Dacryocystorhinostomy is the operation of choice for the prevention of recurrence of dacryocystitis.
* A cutaneous horn of eyelid is frequently associated with an underlying dysplastic (actinic keratisis) or neoplastic (squamous cell carcinoma).
* Operations for ptosis ameliorate the condition but seldom give perfect result.
* The orbital spaces are five in number.

* Simultaneous thrombosis of both cavernous sinuses, with proptosis and disc swelling occurs in diseases of the sphenoid sinuses.
* Optic atrophy is seen in mucocele of the sphenoid sinus.
* The functional efficiency of lacrimal drainge may be assessed by instilling radioactive tracer into conjunctiva and visualizing the gamma camera.
* Most of the orbital veins drain into the superior ophthalmic vein.
* **Grey line** on the inter-marginal strip indicates a tissue plane between orbicularis palpebrum and tarsus.
* The most helpful investigation in the provisional diagnosis of a bilateral proptosis in an infant is abdominal examination.
* Upper lid proptosis with sclerosis of orbit is diagnostic of meningioma.
* The investigation of choice in carotico-cavernous fistula is carotid angiography (but not orbital venography).
* Sebaceous cell carcinoma of the eyelid arises usually from the Meibomian glands.
* Enlargement of the optic canal is typically seen in optic nerve glioma.
* **Kronlein's operation** refers to Orbitotomy.
* Glioma of the optic nerve arises from astrocytes and Oligodendroglial cells of optic nerve.
* Intermittent proptosis occurs in orbital varix.
* Down's syndrome is associated with epicanthus.
* The first sign of cavernous sinus thrombosis is restriction of ocular movements.
* Blepharitis acaria is caused by Demodex folliculorum.
* The most useful technique in assessing the function of the canaliculus is Radioscintillography.
* Congenital hydrocephalus shows **'setting-sun' sign.**
* Antimongoloid obliquity is seen in Crouzon's syndrome where as mongoloid obliquity is seen in Down's syndrome.
* Meningioma affecting orbit most typically arise from optic nerve sheath and lateral portion of the sphenoid ridge.

* A chronic unilateral condition caused by infection with **Actinomyces israeli, C. albicans** and **Aspergillus** species causing a secondary purulent unilateral conjunctivitis that frequently escapes etiological diagnosis is **Canaliculitis.**

* A common condition of ageing characterised by redundancy and loss of elasticity of skin such that a skin fold covers the tarsal portion of the eyelids is known as **Dermatochalasis.**

* An acquired unilateral condition characterised by excessive tearing while eating occurs as a sequalae to Bell's palsy is called **Paradoxic Lacrimation ("Crocodile tears").**

* The technique of radiographic visualisation of the lacrimal duct after the injection of a radio opaque contrast medium into the lumen is **Dacryocystography.**

* Chalazion seldom subsides spontaneously.

GRAVES' DISEASE — EXTERNAL EYE SIGNS

*	Ballet's sign	— Complete immobility of the globe
*	Boston's sign	— Jerky movement of upper lid on downward gaze.
*	Dalrymple's sign	— Staring appearance
*	Emroth's sign	— Puffy swelling of lids
*	Gifford's sign	— Difficulty in everting upper eyelids.
*	Jellineck's sign	— Increased pigmentation of lids
*	Joffroy's sign	— Absence of forehead wrinkling on upward gaze
*	Kocher's sign	— Increased lid retraction with visual fixation
*	Mobius sign	— Difficulty in converging
*	Rosenbach's sign	— Tremor of closed lids
*	Sainton's sign	— Delayed forehead wrinkling after upward gaze
*	Stellwag's sign	— Weakness of fixation on lateral gaze
*	von Graefe's sign	— Upper lid lag on downward gaze

* Miliary tuberculosis may involve any portion of uvea, but choroid is most common.

* The major cause of blindness in leprosy is iritis.

* Pseudoglioma is produced by toxocariasis, tuberculosis and retrolental fibroplasia.

* Ciliary muscle is always paralysed in diphtheria.

* The disease causing angioid streaks are Sickle cell disease, Paget's disease and Ehlers Danlos syndrome.

* **'Pie in the sky'** type field defect is seen in lesion of temporal lobe radiation.

* Ocular manifestations of tuberculosis include phlyctenulosis, Koeppe's nodules broad posterior synechia and mutton fat KPs.

* Deficiency of thiamine vitamin leads to external ophthalmoplegia.

* Alzheimer's disease is associated with visual impairment, inability to read, spatial deficits, bumping into objects and difficulty in recognizing faces.

* **Cotton-wool spots** indicate systemic disease (even a single isolated cotton-wool spot may be an indication of systemic disease).

* In all cases of **Eale's disease,** it is routine to exclude systemic tuberculosis.

* Retina is the sole portion of body where vasculature is available for observation.

* SLE ocular signs are marginal corneal degeneration, episcleritis and scleritis, retinal haemorrhages and cotton-wool retinal exudates.

* Scleromalacia perforans is seen in rheumatoid arthritis.

* **Snowflake deposits** are seen in the edges of cornea in onchocerciasis.

* Optic neuritis is common in myxoedema.

* Acute conjunctivitis is common in measles.

* Ganciclovir is the drug of choice for cytomegalic inclusion retinitis.

* Polyarteritis nodosa causes retinal arteritis.

* Anticholinergics may cause blurred vision in presbyopic patient.

* Symptoms and signs of vitamin A deficiency do not occur until the blood level drops below **50 IU/L.**

* A sudden onset of diplopia with normal pupil in a diabetic patient denotes **extra ocular muscle palsy.**

* Direct invasion from lacrimal adenocarcinoma or carcinoma of the paranasal sinuses and nasopharynx will produce proptosis and ophthalmoplegia which is known as **orbital apex syndrome (Involvement of cranial nerves II, III, IV at the orbital fissure).**

* The most common ocular complication of mumps is **Dacryoadenitis.**

* The type of leprosy commonly associated with ocular symptoms is **Lepromatous Leprosy.**

* The ocular complication when minor tranquilisers are taken regularly is **decreased tear production of lacrimal gland.**

* Optic neuropathy may be seen in pernicious anaemia.

* Acute leukaemia causes haemorrhage in the nerve fibre layer of retina.

* Iridocyclitis is common in Juvenile diabetes.

* **Endophytic tumour** retinoblastoma—grows into vitreous.

* **Exophytic tumour** retinoblastoma—grows in subretinal space (causes retinal detachment).

* Orbital optic nerve tumors in children are most often due to glioma (pilocytic astrocytomas).

* Enucleation is **contraindicated** unless the eye is painful in metastatic ocular carcinoma.

* Retinoblastoma almost never occurs in microphthalmic eyes or those with cataract, except in very rare cases in which a regressed retinoblastoma was observed in a phthisical eye.

* Intervention is not indicated in infantile orbital or lid haemangiomas unless they are causing visual problems.

* The **earliest** clinical feature of orbital extension of the basal-cell carcinoma of the eyelid is diplopia.

* More than 95% of all eyelid basal cell carcinomas that do not involve orbit or bone are less than 20 mm.

* Leukocoria, strabismus and inflammation are the initial signs of retinoblastoma in over 75% of cases.

* The presence of extensive yellow exudate, peripheral telangiectasia and proliferative vitreoretinopathy exclude the diagnosis of retinoblastoma.

* CT scan is the most useful noninvasive ancillary diagnostic test in patient suspected of having a retinoblastoma (more than 90% of retinoblastoma contain calcium).

* In retinoblastoma less than 5 mm thick calcification may not be evident on CT and extraocular retinoblastoma does not calcify.

* Almost all children with metastatic orbital neuroblastoma have bone involvement with diffuse orbital, bone and brain metastasis demonstrable on either CT scan or MRI.

* Most patients with optic nerve gliomas initially present with decreased vision and field loss.

* Ciliary body melanomas causes disturbance of ciliary muscle function, distortion of the lens and displacement of the lens.

* IOP in a patient of late stage of malignant melanoma of choroid is likely to be high and is due to infilteration of the angle by malignant cells, obstruction of venous channels and narrow of AC (due to pushing forward of iris lens diaphragm).

* Ultrasound is best used to diagnose melanoma in late stages.

* Malignant melanoma of ciliary body presents late.

* Metastasis from retinoblastoma first spread to preauricular lymphnode.

* **Lisch nodules** are found on the iris of prepubertal children suffering from von Recklinghausen's disease.

* Malignant melanoma of the uvea does not cause metastasis.

* Secondaries in choroid are usually from breast cancer.

* Intraocular tumour with calcification is characteristic of the retinoblastoma. The indication of retinoblastoma is when it recurs after enucleation and when it is found in the orbit while doing enucleation.

* Malignant melanoma in the iris is rare.

* **Retinoblastoma is usually multicentric.**

* Melanocytic nevi of the eyelids are mostly congenital.

* Sebaceous gland carcinomas of the eyelid are potentially fatal neoplasms.

* Metastatic orbital tumor masses are rarely removed surgically.

* Carcinoma involving this part of eye has the highest incidence of any malignant ocular tumour is **Carcinoma of lid (42%)**.

* The most frequent site of secondary or metastatic ocular malignancies is the **Choroid.**

* This investigation may be very useful in detecting orbital and intraocular masses, especially when visibility with an opthalmoscope is poor (as occurs when cataract is present) is **Ultrasonography.**

* The eponymous name for angiomatosis retinae is **Von Hippel-Lindau Disease.**

* Benign and malignant medullo epitheliomas are tumors that may arise from the **Ciliary body epithelium.**

* Treatment of recurrences in carcinoma of the conjunctiva is **Re-excision.**

* Lactic dehydrogenase activity if raised in aqueous relative to the serum level is suggestive of **Retinoblastoma.**

* Asymptomatic circumscribed choroidal haemangiomas require no treatment.

* Reticulum cell sarcoma is a non-Hodgkin's B-cell lymphoma.

* Leukocoria is the most common mode of presentation in retinoblastoma.

* Children with bilateral retinoblastoma present earlier than those with unilateral involvement.

* Metastatic tumours to the choroid are probably more common than primary malignancies.

* The common sites of rupture of the globe are the **limbus,** the **equator,** and especially **under the rectus muscles,** where the sclera is thinnest.

* The indication of early surgical intervention in traumatic cataract is secondary glaucoma.

* Prolapsed iris in perforating trauma should not be replaced because it will carry intra-ocular infection.
* Open sky vitrectomy is indicated in large intraocular foreign body.
* Prodromal symptoms of sympathetic ophthalmia are photophobia and indistinctness of near objects.
* Injury to the ciliary body region of eye has highest risk of sympathetic ophthalmia.
* A piece of glass in AC is exceptionally difficult to see because of its transparency and refractive index differs little from surrounding media.
* The most distressing sequelae of chemical burns in eye is symblepharon.
* The indication of extraction of lens dislocated into the vitreous is by onset of phacolytic glaucoma and phacoanaphylaxis.
* A non-magnetic foreign body in the vitreous or retina is removed by paraplana vitrectomy followed by removal by viterous forceps.
* Symblepharon formation after caustic injury to the eyes is best prevented by contact lens.
* Perforating injury of the eyes is dangerous because of introduction of infection, post-traumatic iridocyclitis and dreaded symphathetic ophthalmitis.
* Conjunctival foreign body most often gets lodged in upper sulcus subtarsalis.
* In siderosis bulbi the iron after getting electrolytically dissociated gets combined with the cellular proteins of the cell, thus killing the cells and causing atrophy.
* Pathognomonic sign of retained intraocular foreign body is a hole in the iris.
* The **earliest** sign of sympathetic ophthalmia in the uninjured eye is K.P.
* The rupture of the globe occurs at its weakest part in blunt trauma in the neighbourhood of canal of schlemm.
* Following corneal injury spectacles for correcting astigmatism should be prescribed after **six weeks.**

* **Vossius's ring** is the impairment of the contracted pupil on the anterior surface of the lens in blunt trauma of eye.

* Post-traumatic glaucoma is due to ghost cell obstruction, iridocyclitis and phacolytic glaucoma.

* Sympathetic ophthalmitis in the sympathizing eye is almost always acute plastic iridocyclitis.

* The treatment of established sympathetic ophthalmitis in the uninjured eye is systemic and topical steroids.

* The best method of discovering a foreign body is to open the cornea is Bio-microscopy after florescein staining.

* The **earliest** symptom of sympathetic ophthalmia is photophobia.

* Sympathetic ophthalmia is extremely rare if actual suppuration has occurred in exciting eye.

* In blunt trauma of the eye ball with the force coming from down and out the sclera ruptures supero-nasally.

* Liquor ammonia causes maximum damage to the cornea.

* In concussion cataract fine tears in the lens capsule occurs at posterior pole of the lens.

* Prolapsed iris through corneal lacerations are best treated by excision.

* A globule of oil in anterior chamber is the look seen in anterior dislocation of the lens.

* Foreign bodies are the most frequent cause of eye injury.

* Tetanus prophylaxis is indicated whenever penetrating injury in eye occurs.

* Partial tear of suspensory ligament may lead to subluxation.

* An irregularity of the corneal surface due to a minute abrasion laceration or foreign body may be demonstrated by instillation of **Sterile fluroscein.**

* Routine instillation of a topical anaesthetic for pain in abrasions of cornea and conjunctiva is contraindicated because **delays normal healing of the epithelium.**

* Any injury severe enough to cause intraocular haemorrhage involves the danger of delayed secondary haemorrhage from a damaged uveal vessel, which may cause **Intractable glaucoma (and permanent damage to eyeball).**

* Persons using the hallucinogenic drugs such as LSD have been particularly prone to **Solar macular burns.**

* An electromagnetic detecting device for localisation of metalic foreign bodies is **Berman metal locator.**

* In the concussion injuries due to gunshot wounds, a rupture of the retina is associated with a similar rupture of the choroid and such cases shows a characteristic picture of **traumatic proliferating chorioretinopathy.**

* Optic nerve is not frequently injured in fractures of the base of the skull.

* Post-traumatic iridocyclitis is a common sequel to a perforating wound.

Sutures :

* *8/0 Gauge silk*—> closure of corneo-scleral or scleral wounds.

* *5/0 or 6/0 silk*—> to close skin incisions around eye.

* *4/0 Gauge silk (thicker)*—> to retract the lids & skin flaps; to pass beneath rectus muscle and to rotate globe.

* *10/0 Nylon (Monofilament)*—> is nonabsorable, least reaction, no scarring (ideal suture material).

* *10/0*—> is ideal for suturing cornea (under microscope).

* 5/0 Dacron non-absorbable; multifilament, Polyester—>for high tensile strength (eg. suturing of implants to sclera in retinal detachment operation).

* *6/0 Catgut & Collagen*—> absorbable, more reaction & used ideally for closure of conjunctival and Tenon's capsule, retachment of ocular muscles.

* Preplaced sutures are inserted before lens removal in cataract surgery.

* Bilateral proptosis is caused by Crouzon's disease.

* The safe anaesthesia for intraocular surgery is peribulbar anaesthesia.

* **O'Brien facial nerve block** with 2 cc of 2% novocaine is injected on the neck of the mandible just below the condyle to paralyse orbicularis muscle.

* The absolute indications for enucleation is sympathetic ophthalmia and malignancy of the globe.

* To give **'Ciliary ganglion block'** the needle is to be pushed from the junction of middle third and lateral third of inferior orbital margin—>upwards, backwards and medially towards the apex of the orbit (the patient must be asked to look upwards during the injection).

* Balanced salt solution is used to carry out irrigation of AC in extracapsular cataract extraction.

* Extracapsular extraction (ECCE) is indicated in immature cortical, nuclear, postcortical and hypermature sclerotic cataracts.

* The percentage of corneal graft acceptance is high because of avascularity of cornea.

* Discission (needling) operation is indicated for congenital cataract, traumatic cataract in children and any cataract below the age of 24 years.

* Paracentesis of AC may be employed as a part of treatment in hyphaema with ↑ IOP.

* Risk of vitreous loss is present in ICCE.

* In ECCE, there is no risk of vitreous loss because of intact posterior capsule.

* If the patient is an young adult, chymotrypsin is used in intracapsular cataract extraction.

* The surgery which most suits to a patient of unilateral traumatic cataract in a young adult is extracapsular cataract extraction with intra-ocular implantation.

* Intermittent proptosis occurs in orbital varix.

* The most important indication for extracapsular extraction of lens is subluxated lens.

* Healon or methylcellulose is used in cataract surgery/keratoplasty to protect endothelium of the cornea.

* Ciliary block lowers the IOP and makes the iris painles during iridectomy.

* Paracentesis is a temporary measure for secondary glaucoma (due to acute iridocyclitis, Burst Morgagnian cataract, Corneal ulcer with Hypopyon, threatened perforation of a corneal ulcer and severe hyphaema).

* The **most safe site** of fixation of the intraocular lens is endocapsular.

* Anterior sclerotomy is a fistulising operation for temporary period only (for epidemic dropsy).

* Radial keratotomy is carried out to treat patient of myopia.

* In ECCE, there is always a chance of after cataract formation.

* Iridencleisis operation indications are like those of trephining operation and can also be done for acute congestive glaucoma.

* In extracapsular cataract extraction the part of the lens left behind is posterior capsule.

* Sutures should always be used in cataract surgery.

* Preliminary iridectomy is a complete iridectomy at 12 O' clock position.

* Epikeratophakia is **contraindicated** in lagophthalmos.

* The eponymous name for cauterization of the sclera with a peripheral iridectomy, simple glaucoma operation is **"Scheie's thermosclerectomy"**.

* Mc Reynold's operation is indicated for **progressive pterygium.**

* **Jensen's procedure** is used to improve abduction in cases of 6th nerve palsy and is combined with a recession of the medial rectus muscle.

* In **automated vitrectomy** procedure the vitreous is excised from the AC with the Kaufman vitrector.

* **Radial Keratotomy (RK)** decreases myopia by flattening the cornea

* Paracentesis is a temporary measure for secondary glaucoma.

* Cyclodialysis is indicated in aphakic glaucoma.

* Striate keratitis is a complication following extraction of lens.

* **Blindness**—Corrected visual acuity of 6/60 (20/200) or less in the better eye, or a visual field of no more than 20 degrees in the better eye.

* **Visually handicapped**—Visual acuity in the better eye is 6/18 or less.
* **Economical blindness**—Visual acuity in better eye is 6/60 or less and visual field is restricted to 20°.
* **Legal blindness**—Loss of vision sufficient to prevent one from being self-supporting in an occupation, making the individual dependent on other persons, agencies, or devices in order to live.
* At extremely high illuminations the visual acuity diminishes.
* The conjunctival epithelium in Vitamin A deficiency is transformed from normal columnar to stratified squamous (with a resultant loss of goblet cells, formation of granular cell layer & keratinization of the surface).
* The criteria of blindness in Great Britain is a visual acuity in the better eye of 3/60 where as in United States, Canada and WHO is 6/60.
* In right handed people the source of light while writing should come from behind and left side.
* Night blindness sometimes termed as 'Chicken eyes' (because chicken lack rods and are thus night blind).
* Xerophthalmia is a medical emergency as it carries a high risk of corneal destruction and blindness; sepsis and death.
* When scarring is severe in trachoma, blindness results.
* Blinded adults learn Braille less easily than children.
* Most color blind people have normal visual acuity.
* Decreased visual acuity in one eye in the absence of any organic eye disease responsible for the visual impairment is known as **Amblyopia ("Lazy eye").**
* Disturbances of vision with conjunctivitis and photophobia which are normally temporary conditions only caused by exposing the eyes to the glare of the sun on snow is called **Snow blindness.**
* Rapid loss of vision, going on to complete blindness occurring in some cases of approaching uraemia and of cortical origin is termed as **Bright's blindness.**
* **Commonest** cause of acquired anomaly of colour vision is diabetic retinopathy.

* Glare may be regarded as light in the wrong place.
* Most common primary benign tumor of orbit is :
  * In infant and children—Capillary Hemangioma
  * In adult—Cavernous Hemangioma.
* **Chocolate Cysts** of orbit is encysted blood in lymphangiomas.
* Demostration of cross striations in the tumor cells is **pathognomonic** of Rhabdomysarcoma.
* **"Racquet Cells"** or **"Strap Cells"** are characteristic of **embryonal** form of rhabdomyosarcoma.
* **Most malignant** type of Rhabdomyosarcoma is alveolar type.
* **Rarest** type and having best **prognosis** of rhabdomyosarcoma is pleomorhic type.
* Tumor which is a expansile & reducible and forms a gap in the underlying bone of orbit is Meningo-Encephalocele.
* Complex choriostoma has a peculiar association with the Linear Sebaceous Nevus of Jadassohn.
* Small sessile sq. papilloma of conjunctiva can be treated with **topical corticosteroid.**
* Invasive squamous cell carcinoma of conjunctiva usually occurs as **natural extension** of CIN. (Conjunctival Intraepithelial Neoplasia) through the basement membrane.
* Pyogenic Granuloma of the conjunctiva is neither pyogenic **nor** granulomatous but a proliferative fibrovascular response to prior tissue insult by inflammation, surgery or non-surgical trauma.
* **"Chocolate Cysts"** of conjunctiva is conjunctival lymphangioma.
  * Breast carcinoma in female
  * Cutaneous melanoma in male
* Naevus flammeus is a capillary hemangioma.
* Advanced retinoblastoma is the retinoblastoma with :
  * Extraocular extension or
  * Optic nerve invasion

* **Specific** histologic finding of retinoblastoma :
  * Flexner-Wintersteiner rosette
  * Fleurettes
* Most widely used staging system of retinoblastoma is :**Reeseellisworth classification.**
* Most helpful and **sensitive** diagnostic test for retinoblastoma is CT-scan (next best method is Ultrasonography).
* The mainstay of conservative therapy of retinoblastoma is, external beam radiotherapy.
* Most **radioresistant** structure in the eye is sclera.
* TOC in retinoblastoma, when tumor fills most of the globe and having very little or no hope of vision is Enucleation.
* Most important factor to consider in enucleation in case of retinoblastoma is to obtain a long stump of optic nerve.
* **Cryotherapy** is useful for small tumor anterior to the equator when the tumor is mostly confined to the sensory retina.
* **Contraindications of cryotherapy :**
  * Significant vitreous seeding.
  * Tumors greater than 5 mm. in diameter and greater than 2.5 mm in thickness.
* TOC of small retinoblastoma in the posterior pole is xenon photocoagulation.
* Radioprotectors are used to protect normal cells from hazards of ionising radiation. These include :
  * WR-2721 (Ethiofos)
  * WR-77913
* **Trilateral retinoblastoma** consists of bilateral retinoblastoma with midline intracranial tumor (most commonly Pineal Gland tumors).
* Retinoma or retinocytoma is benign variant of retinoblastoma.
* Calcification is an important diagnostic feature of the endophytic retinoblastoma.
* A higher prevalence of retinoblastoma is reported with :
  * Tirsomy -21
  * Delection of long arm of the D-chromosome.

* **CEA** (carcinoembryonic antigen) may be elevated in retinoblastoma.
* **"Cluster of Grapes"** appearance is characteristic of cavernous hemangioma of the retina.

Indications of botulinum toxin in opthalmology

A. **Guidelines for the use of B otulinum Toxin in Strabismus**
   1. Investigation of binocular states
   2. VI nerve palsy - Ac/chr
   3. III nerve palsy (partly recovery)
   4. IV nerve palsy (chronic)
   5. Thyroid strabismus
   6. Strabismus after retinal detachment
   7. Surgical over correction
   8. Oscillopsia

B. **Facial movement disorder**
   — Blepharespasm-Treatment of choice
   — Hemifacial spasm-in selected cases
   — Hemifacial synkinesis- Treatment of choice

C. **Ptosis indn**
   — Indolent corneal ulceration
   — Ac. facial Nerve pales esp with
   — Corneal anaesthesia
   — Absent Bell's phenomenon
   — Ocular motor palsy

D. **Others**
   — Periocular skin wrinkles (crow's feet)
   — Orbicularis muscle weakness

* Fibres of Gudden's commissure are found in medial root of optic tract.
* Base curves of a lens can be checked by Geneva lens measure.
* On accommodation the lenticular changes are - anterior pole moves forward, physiological lenticonus and lens moves inferiorly.

* **'Critical period'** for visual acquity in humans begins at approximately 4 months.
* **Cotton wool spot** mainly results due to infarction.
* **Collier's sign** is seen in midbrain disease.
* The resonances in brain which cause apparent increase in brightness is known as **Broca Sulza effect.**
* **'Key hole'** optic foramen is encountered as a congenital anomaly in 4% people and may be unilateral.
* Inferolateral border of optic canal is called "optic strut".
* **"J-shaped"** sella is also known as **'omega shaped'**, **'shoe-shaped'**,**'hour-glass sella'** and represent an exaggeration of the normal slight impression of the sulcus chiasmaticus.
* Pseudodendrites are associated with soft contact lens wear.
* **Krukenberg's spindle** is due to melanin.
* **Salzman's nodular degeneration** in cornea occurs following trachoma.
* **Jones test** is used for evaluating lacrimal function.
* **Siegrist's spots** are seen in choroiditis.
* **Stockers's lines** are due to iron.
* **Sursumversion** is elevation of both eyes.
* **Titmus test** is done for stereoacquity.
* Aqueous flare is an example of **Tyndall effect.**
* Viers rod is used for canalicular lacerations.
* **Most common** cause of iridoplegia is trauma.
* Glands of Manz are found in conjunctiva.
* **Circle of Zinn-Haller** is found by anastomosis of branches of short posterior ciliary arteries.
* **Barkan's membrance** (extending from schwalbe's line over the angle) is seen in congenital glaucoma.
* On fundoscopy, double angulation of blood vessels as they dive sharply backwards and then turn along the steep wall of the excavation before angling again into the floor of the cup is a common but not necessarily a pathognomonic sign in primary angle closure glaucoma, is also called **Bayonetting sign.**

* Asteriod hyalosis is also called Benson's disease.

* **Terson's syndrome** is in which a patient with subarachnoid bleed develops a vitreous haemorrge.

* IV (trochlear) nerve is the **longest** and most slender of all cranial nerves. It is the only cranial nerve to emerge from the dorsal aspect of the brain. It is the only completely crossed cranial nerve.

* **Bielschawskly test** is used to detect IV cranial nerve palsy.

* Glaucomatocyclitic crisis is also known as **Posnner-Schlossman syndrome.**

* **Salus sign** is seen in grade 2 hypertensive retinopathy

* Bonnet's sign and gunn's sign are seen in grade 3 hypestensive retinopathy

* Visual threshold increases as the subject moves from absolute darkness to very bright sunlight by a factor of 12 log unit

* Sclera is pierced by **three** groups of apertures

* Scleral collagen is mainly of type I and type III type IV collagen is found in the lamina cribrosa which is the **weakest** past of sclera

* **Fluff balls** are seen in anterior vitreous in fungal endophthalmitis (seen about 8 days following surgery)

* **Corneal pigmentation**

* **Hassall-Henle warts** are peripheral excrescences in Descemet's membrane, that are frequently seen in elderly individuals.

* **Honey comb pattern** on examination is seen in Reis-Buckler's dystrophy.

* 15% patients cured of bilateral retinoblastoma will develop an unrelated neoplasm later in life (most commonly osteosarcoma of femur).

* **Mulberry like appearance** is seen in retinal astrocytomas.

* The inner segment of the photoreceptor consists of an outer portion named the 'ellipsoid', rich in mitochondria and an inner portion, the 'myoid', rich in components for protein synthesis.

* Ganglion cells do not exist at fovea or optic disc

* **'Twitch sign'** of Cogan (elicited by asking the patient to rapidly redirect his gaze from the downward to the primary position when the upper lid will be seen to twitch upward and then slowly resettle to its ptosis position).

* Anterior chamber of IOL's have designs of Choyce Mark VIII and IX, Kelman, Leiske flexible and Mcghah late flex. Iris supported IOL's are Binkhorst 4 loop, Federor Sputnik and worst medallion. Iridocapsular supported IOL is Binhorst 2 loop. Posterior chamber IOL's are Shearing, Simcoe, Sinskey, Sheets and Anis. Rigid posterior chamber IOL are Boberg Ans and Severin.

* UGH syndrome consists of uveitis, glaucoma and hyphema, is more common with angle-supported IOL's than other designs.

* **Irvine Gass syndrome** is cystoid maculopathy, more common with anterior chamber lenses.

* Scleritis is frequently associated with rheumatoid arthritis.

* Swollen eyelids may indicate endocrine disorder, general oedema or simple ageing.

* Ptosis is frequently a hereditary disease.

* Children do not grow out of a true squint.

* Cranial arteritis can lead to ischemic pupillopathy.

* An anaesthetic red eye should be investigated for corneal abrasion or glaucoma.

* Unilateral high myopia may cause pseudoproptosis

* Hypothyroidism is typified by oedema of lower lids and watering eyes.

* Central retina contains a yellow pigment, xanthophyll

* **Sheridan-Gardener test** is used to measure the visual acquity of young children (or illiterate patients)

* In occlusion of central retinal vein, loss of vision is first noticed on walking.

* Upbeat nystagmus is due to cerebellar lesion whereas downbeat is due to lesions at the level of foramen magnum

* Fresh KP's are white and round whereas old KP's tend to shrink, fade and become pigmented.

* Type A spindle cell tumors (choroidal melanomas) have best prognosis whereas epitheloid cell type has the worst prognosis.

* In fascicular type choroidal melanoma, cells are arranged in a palisading or ribbon like arrangement.

* **'Chocolate cysts'** are seen in lymphangioma of orbit

* **Jenson's choroiditis** refers to a focal, often sectoral, retinitis adjacent to optic nerve head.

* **'Egg-yolk' lesions** are seen in stage 4 (vitelliruptive) of Best's macular degeneration.

* In **Ghost cells glaucoma**, there is obstruction to aqueous out flow due to degenerate and less pliable red blood cells (which turn into ghost cells).

* Inner mucin layer of tear is formed by goblet cells and glands of Manz and crypts of Henle.

* **Sea saw nystagmus of Maddox** is seen in pituitary adenoma. **Double floor sign** is also seen an X-ray skull.

* **Double ring sign** is seen in optic nerve hypoplasia.

* **Flying corpuscle test** is used in macular disease.

* **Glass blowers cataract** is caused by infrared energy and is characterized by `scroll' of peeled anterior lens capsule.

* Glaucomflecken are small, grey-white anterior capsular or capsular opacities seen in pupillary region, which are diagnostic of a previous acute congestive glaucoma attack.

* Microspherophakia is the main ocular feature of hyperlysinemia.

* **Haab's striae** are seen in dislocated lens in buphthalmos.

* **Panum's space** (area) of single binocular vision is a zone about the horopter in which objects are seen singly. Objects in front of or behind Panum's space are seen double. This is the basis of physioloigcal diplopia.

* *Hering's law* states that during any conjugate eye movement, equal and simultaneous innervation flows to the yoke muscles.

* **Hermansky-Pudlak syndrome** consists of a triad of albinism, haemorrhagic diathesis and ceroid-lipofuscin storage.

* **Hollenhorst's plaques** (cholesterol emboli) are usually due to necrosis and ulceration of an atheromatous plaque with discharge of its contents into the circulation.

* P50 is abnormal in the presence of macular disease, however P50/N95 ratio is normal.

* Brown pigmented eyes show a reduced ocular hypotensive response to pilocarpine than blue eyes due to pigment binding.

* Acetazolamide produces myopia due to shallowing of ant. chamber secondary to forward shift of lens.

* Eyestrain is a collective term for a ocular discomfort and associated symptoms, possibly aggravated by the intense use of eyes. The main causes are small refractive error, inadequate accommodative power and muscle imbalance between the two eyes.

* Posterior uveitis, choroiditis, may affect vision if it involves the central retina.

* Chronic simple glaucoma may go unnoticed by patient if it affects only the peripheral field.

* The presence of pigmented granules in the anterior vitreous (**tobacco dust**) is strongly suggestive of the presence of the retinal tear.

* A round opacity *hyaloid ring* representing the annular attachment of the vitreous cortex to the optic disc may be seen in mid or posterior vitreous in post. vitreous detachment.

* Applanation Tonometer is based on the **Imbert Fick law** which states that for an ideal, dry, thin-walled sphere the pressure inside the sphere (P) equals the force necessary to flatten its surface divided by the area of flattening (P=F/A).

* **Jones primary dye test** differentiates a watering due to partial obstruction of lacrimal passages from primary hypersecretion of tears.

* **Fundus albipunctatus** is rare condition characterized by congenital stationary night blindness. It is autosomal dominant or recessive and ophthalmologic examination shows yellow-white spots.

* **Kearns-Sayre syndrome** consists of ocular myopathy with ptosis and heart block.
* **Kocher's sign** Staring and frightened appearance of eyes which is particularly marked on attentive fixation.
* Lens absorbs short wave length blue/UV light.
* Alpha, beta and gamma crystallins are the only crystallins found in humans. **Alpha crystallin** has been found in heart, brain and lung. Beta crystallin is the most common crystallin in lens (55%) followed by alpha (35%) and gamma (10%). Gamma crystallins are found mainly in the central core lesion.
* Chlorpromazine is the only phenothiazine implicated in causing cataract.
* Age-related liquefaction of vitreous begins in the central part and by the age of 50, upto 25% of individuals have a significant degree of liquefaction.
* **Krimsky test** is used to detect strabismus.
* **Molteno and Krupin-Denver valves** are used in advanced neovascular glaucoma.
* **Lacquer cracks** are seen in myopic macutopathy.
* **Lamellar dot sign** (indicating that in meridia, neural tissue destruction), is seen in acute congestive glaucoma.
* **Peau d' orange** or pigmentary retinal mottling is seen in **angioid streaks**.
* **Plateau Iris syndrome** is a rare cause of acute glaucoma which occurs in an eye in which iris is inserted anteriorly on the ciliary body. Treatment is miotics and not peripheral iridectomy.
* **Pseudoretinitis pigmentosa** is seen in trauma, inflammation (syphilis, rubella, Vogt Koyangi Harada syndrome, toxicity by chloroquine), or phenothiazines (CPZ, thioridazine), vascular (occlusion of ophthalmic artery), spontaneous retinal detachment.
* **Pseudomacular holes** are caused by defects in an epiretinal membrane covering fovea.
* **Pulfrich's phenomenon** is another feature of optic nerve disorder in which depth perception particularly for moving objects is impaired.

* **Vogt's limbal girdle** is seen in healthy elderly patients and consists of white irregular nasal and temporal deposits at the limbus.

* **Three quarters** of tear volume is eliminated by lacrimal drainage system, **one quarter** is evaporated. Of that **two thirds** is drained by lower canaliculus and **one third** by the upper canaliculus.

* **Myokymia** (fibrillary twitching of eyelids) is seen commonly due to irritation within the VII nerve. It is often idiopathic, but is associated with fatigue, thyrotoxicosis, stress and refractive errors.

* **Lambert's law** states that when a parallel beam of light falls on a semitransparent, hemogeneous substance, the intensity of the transmitted light decreases exponentially as distance through the substance increases.

* **Beer's law** states that if a parallel beam of light is transmitted a known substance through a clear solution with a dissolved solute, the intensity of the transmitted light decreases expenentially as the concentration of solute increases.

* A substance which emits light of a certain wavelength at a given temperature can also absorb light of the same wavelength at that temperature. This is called **Kirchhoff's law.**

* Buphthalmos (or infantile glaucoma) usually affects both eyes.

* Mycotic corneal ulcer is most often caused by Aspergillus fumigatus : marginal corneal ulcer is usually caused by Koch-weeks bacillus, Hypopyon ulcer is usually caused by Pneumococous.

* Mooren's ulcer never perforates the cornea.

* Retrobulbar anaesthesia causes fall in IOP.

* In addition to vitamin A deficiency. night blindness may be seen in Retinitis pigmentosa, Glaucoma, Oguchi's disease, Chorioderma etc.

* Cornea, lens and vitreous are avascular structures of eye.

* 1.4% saline is isotonic with tear.

* Detached retina gives blue colour in fundus.

* Earliest change of diabetic retinopathy is microaneurysms whereas most detectable is venous abnormalities and most specific is hard exudates.

* Anatomical rest position of eye is exopheric state.
* Devic's disease or neuromyelitis optica is paralysis of extra ocular muscles.
* Berlin's oedema or commotio retinae results due to blow to eye.
* **Gaule's spots** are related to neuroparalytic keratitis.
* **Salu's sign** is deflection of retinal vein alongwith concealment.
* 'Blaskowicz operation" is done for Ptosis.
* Chronic dacryocystitis is more common in women.
* Guanethidine is used for the treatment of cataract.
* "Protanopes" can not see red.
* "Deuteroanopes" can not see green.
* The brown ring seen on the anterior surface of lens in cases of blunt injury is known as **"Vossius ring"**.
* The pigmented ring seen in the cornea in Wilson's disease is known as **Kayser-Flischer ring.**
* The pigmented ring seen in the corneal ulcer.
* The zone of greatest sensibility in the cornea is small area in the centre of the cornea.
* "Keratometer" is useful for determining the corneal curvature.
* Visual angle is defined as the angle substended by an object at nodal point.
* The optical axis of the eye passes through centre of lens and centre of cornea.
* Visual axis of eye passes through nodal point, macula and fixation point.
* The angle between visual axis and optical axis is called **"angle alpha"**.
* The angle between optical axis and fixation axis is called **"angle gamma"**.
* The angle between central pupillary line and visual axis is called **"angle kappa"**.
* The eye is normally hypermetropic for red rays.
* The eye is normally myopic for blue rays.
* Central serous retinopathy usually occurs in young male.

* Superficial retinal haemorrhages usually occur in young male.

* Subhyaloid haemorrhages usually occur in the neighbourhood of macula.

* The retina is initially white in cases of central retinal artery occlusion.

* **"Cattle-truck appearance"** is seen in cases of central retinal artery occlusion.

* "Haemorrhagic glucoma" is due to neovascularization of angle.

* **'Groundglass' cornea and 'Salmon pathces'** (on corneas) or interstitial keratitis due to congenital syphilis.

* Keratoconus usually manifests in girls after puberty and contact lens is useful.

* In Argyll-Robertson Pupil, there is no light reflex whereas in inverse type, convergence and accommodation are poor.

* Hutchison's pupil is seen in head injury (dilated immobile pupil on same side).

* In deep sleep, there is bilateral constriction of pupils.

* In iridocyclitis, pain is along branches of V nerve and is worse at night.

* Heterochromic cyclitis of Fuch's has fine KP's no posterior synechia and complicated cataract.

* Cupuliform of posterior cortical cataract never matures.

* **Rosette shaped cataract** is seen in trauma, **snowflake cataract** in diabetes mellitus and **Bread-Crumb** appearance in complicated type.

* Rings of Soemmering and Elscchnig's pearls are seen in aftercataract.

* Massage cataract is dislocated lens developing cataract due to endothelial damage.

* Vitreous never regenerates.

* Applanation tomometer was devised by Goldman in 1954.

* **Earliest sign** of chronic simple glaucoma is cupping of optic disc and *pathognomic sign is* pulsation of retinal arteries at margin of disc. Earliest field defect is baring of blind spot.

* Miotics are not useful in buphthalmos, epidemic dropsy glaucoma, aphakic glaucoma, glaucoma inversus, glaucomatocyclitic crisis (in this mydriatric and surgery also contraindicated).

* Treatment of malignant glaucoma is removal of lens.
* Fovea centralis has no rods (but only cones), no nerve fibre layer and no direct blood vessels.
* **"Soft exudates"** are usually seen in cases of hypertensive retinopathy.
* **Hard exudates** are seen in diabetic retinopathy.
* **"Microaneurysms"** are seen in diabetic retinopathy.
* **"Pepper and salt" fundus** is seen in cases of congenital syphilis.
* Toxoplasmosis usually affects macula.
* Eale's disease is seen in young males.
* Angioid streaks are usually due to break in Bruch's membrane.
* Senile macular degeneration is due to break in Bruch's membrane.
* "Retinal veins" are usually affected in Eale's disease
* **"Tubular vision"** is seen in cases of retinitis pigmentosa.
* In retinitis pigmentosa, Rods are primarily affected.
* **"Index myopia"** occurs in nuclear cataract.
* **"Pseudopapillitis"** is seen in hypermetropia.
* **"Keratoconus"** can be corrected by contact lens.
* **"Fuch's fleck"** is seen in degenerative myopia.
* Central scotoma is **characteristic** of papillitis.
* Malignant glaucoma is produced after surgery.
* Intense itching is the most characteristic feature of spring catarrh.
* Intraocular pressure is best measured by applanation tonometry.
* A dendritic corneal ulcer is typically seen in Herpes simplex infection.
* Steroids are contraindicated in dendritic ulcer.
* Chloroquine therapy may produce characteristic **bull's eye.**
* Placido's disc is used to detect the smoothness or irregularities of corneal surface.
* Corneal thickness is measure by pachometer.
* **Munson's sign** is seen in keratoconus.
* Lenticular rosette formation is usually associated with concussion cataract.
* **"Sun-grain" follicles** are characteristic of trachoma.
* **"Sago-grain" follicles** are characteristic of trachoma.

* Direct ophthalmoscopy reveals virtual, erect and magnified image.
* In indirect ophthalmoscopy, the image is inverted real and magnified.
* Young-Helmholtz has propounded the trichromatic theory of colour vision.
* In a case of aphakia the astigmatism is usually against the rule.
* Irregular astigmatism can best be corrected by hard contact lenses.
* Pleoptics is useful in patient with eccenteric fixation.
* Pleoptics was advocated first of all by **Bangerter.**
* Cyclodialysis is generally performed in aphakic glaucoma.
* Discission is not done in immature cataract.
* Combined lens extraction is extracapsular extraction with complete iridectomy.
* The best indication for erisophake is cataract goufle.
* The most important indication for extracapsular extraction of lens is subluxated lens.
* **"Jaeche-Arlt operation"** is done for Entropion.
* Blind spot corresponds to optic nerve-head where there is no retina.
* **Forester-Fuch's spots** may be the complications of myopia.
* **Commonest** type of myopia is simple or developmental (and not congenital, pathological or degenerative).
* Main symptoms of hypermetropia is headache whereas that of myopia is reduced visual acquity for distance (there is no headache) whereas astigmatism has both headache and reduced acquity.
* Contact lens is useful for irregular astigmatism whereas cylindrical lens is used for regular astigmatism.
* Normal flora of conjunctiva includes Coagulase negative staphylococcus and diphtheroids.
* Gonococcus is main cause of ophthalmia neonatorum which is common in first three weeks of life.
* Angular conjunctivitis is caused by Morax-Axenfield diplobacilus.
* Common named bacteria are — Kochweeks (Haemophillus aegypticus), Kleb Loeffer (Corynebacterium) and Morax Axenfield diplobacillus (Haemophillus lacunatum)

* Folliculosis is more common in lower fornix and Trachoma is more common in upper tarsal conjunctiva and fornix.

* Peritomy is done in trachoma as a treatment for pannus.

* Phlyctena is a compact mass of lymphocytes and polymorphs underneath the epithelium.

* **Cobble stone appearance** (mainly on upper palpebral conjunctiva with no fornix involvement), Ropy secretions, Cauliflower like excresences and **Trantas spots** (in bulbar type) are seen in vernal conjunctivitis or spring catarrh.

* Diphtheria and gonococcus can penetrate normal cornea.

* Central corneal ulcers are mainly exogenous whereas peripheral ones are mainly endogenous.

* Atropine (mydriatics) is the most important drug for treatment of corneal ulcer.

* Commonest cause of corneal opacity is healed corneal ulcer.

* In the eyelid—the **glands of Moll** open between the lashes.

* A **stye** is synonymous with **external hordeolum** is frequently associated with staphylococcal blepharitis; may progress to a chalazion; may be associated with acne rosacea.

* A cyst of Zeis may appear similar to a sweat gland cyst

* A keratoacanthoma may undergo **spontaneous regression.**

* A squamous cell carcinoma grows faster than a basal cell carcinoma.

* In trichiasis corneal pannus is a complication; epilation is an ineffective method of treatment.

* **Districhiasis** is a condition where lashes may grow out or the Meibomian gland orifices.

* **Ectropion** of the involutional type is treated with the **Byron-Smith modification of the Kuhnt-Szymanowski procedure** of the cicatrical type may require treatment with transposition flaps.

* In the upper eyelid, Muller's muscle originates just below **Whitnall's ligament.**

* Anterior PHPV/PFV	Posterior PHPV/PFV

(Persistant Hyperplastic primmary Vitrous / persistent fetal vasculature syndrome)

Abnormality confined to anterior segment and often involves the lens	Abnormality confined to posterior segment and lens is usually clear
* *Typical Presentation* Unilateral Leucocorna	Typical presentation Unilateral Leucocoria, Strabismus, Nystagmus
Signs & complications	*Signs & complications*
* Retrolental mass into which elongated ciliary processes are inserted	* A dense white membrane or a prominent retinal fold extending from the optic disc to ora serrata
* Cataract	
* Shallow Anterior Chamber and angle closure Glaucoma	* Preretinal membrane
	* Tractional Retinal folds and tractional retinal detachment
* Recurrent intraocular hemorrhage	* Retinal dysplasia and optic nerve hypoplasia (may be seen)
	* Microphthalmia
Treatment Vitreoretinal surgery in Selected early cases to salvage vision	Treatment is not possible

* **Disorders that may present with Retinal or Choroidal Dystrophies**

Autosomal Recessive (AR)	Autosomal Dominant (AD)	Variable Inheritance
Macular Dystrophies Dystrophies	**Retinal Macular Dystrophies**	**Retinal Macular Dystrophies**
* Stargardt disease (Juvenile Macular Dystrophy)	* Juvenile Best disease (vitelliform dystrophy)	* Retinitis Pigmentosa (AD/AR/XL)
* Fundus flavimaculatus	* Sorsby pseudoinflammatory macular dystrophy	* Progressive Cone Dystrophy (AR or XL)
* Leber Congenital Amaurosis	* North Carolina macular dystrophy	* Alport syndrome (XLD)
* Bietti Crystallene Dystrophy	* Pattern dystrophy	

* Conditions associated with Retinitis Pigmentosa (Retinal Dystrophy
  -Bassen karnzweigg Syndrome
  -Refsum's Syndrome
  -Kearns Sayre Syndrome
  Bardet Biedl syndrome (Laurence Moon Biedl syndrome)
  - Usher's syndrome
  - Freidreich's ataxia

(Butterfly macular dystrophy)
* Benign concentric annular macular Dystrophy
* Adult vitelliform foveomacular dystrophy
* Familial drusen
* Dominant Cystoid
* Macular Edema

---

* **Proptosis with Orbital Varices**

Features	Orbital Varices	Encephalocele	Carticocavernous Fistula
Pathology/ **Pathogenesis**	Result from weakened orbital venous system that enlarges with increased venous pressure	Results from herniation of intracranial content through a congenital defect at base of skull	Results from an AV fistula between carotid and cavernous sinus usually after head injury
Age of presentation	Early Childhood to late Middle Age	During Infancy	Traumatic : Any age (days or weeks after head injury) Spontaneous Adults/ Elderly
Unilateral/ Bilateral	Unilateral (most cases)		Usually unulateral (ipsilateral) but may be bi lateral or contralateral
Pulsatile/ Compressible	Non pulsatile Compressible	May be pulsatile Reducible but not compressible	Pulsatile
Brui & Thrill	No Brui/No Thrill	No Brul/No thrill	Brui & Thrill present

Precipitatin Factor	As the orbital veins are devoid of valves rapidly reversible proptosis may be precipitated by increasing venous pressure coughing, straining, Valsava manouvre, assuming Dependent Postion external compression of Jugular vein	Cyst increase in size on straining or crying	
MRI/CT	Show Phleboliths (Echogenic shadows)	Show Bony defects responsible for herniation	Prominence of superior ophthalmic vein and diffuse enlargement of extra ocular muscles

* **Proptosis with neurofibromatosis** is not compressible and is not precipitated on increasing venous pressure.

* **Proptosis in Encephalocele** is reducible but not compressible and Echogenic shadows are not a characteristic feature

* **Proptosis in Caroticocavernous Fistula** is pulsatile, associated with Brui and Thrill and is not precipitaed or aggrevated by increasing venous pressure.

* **Transparency of the Cornea :**

1. **Anatomical factors :**

    * Avascularity of cornea

    * Absence of pigment in the cornea

    * Demyelinated nerve supply

    * Regular arrangement of epithelial and endothelial cells.

    * Regular arrangement of stromal collagen fibrils (Lattice theory)

    * Paucity of cells in the stroma

    * Epithelial cells are non-keratinised

    * Anterior surface of the tear film helps in forming a regular refracting surface

2.   **Relative dehydration (de turgescence) of the stroma which is maintained by :**

*   Epithelium, which is **largely** impermeable to water (It must be understood that stroma is not dehydrated, it is in a relative state of dehydration. Stromal water content is 78% and two factors contribute to the prevention of stromal swelling i.e. the endothelial barrier and the pump functions of the endothelium. The barrier is incomplete compared with the epithelial barrier).

*   Endothelial transport system pumps fluid from the corneal stroma to the aqueous by **Na+K+ATPase** mechanism

*   Special inter **cellular junction** in the endothelium is also responsible to control **the fluid** traffic

3.   Intra ocular pressure : Increased I.O.P. leads to endothelial tears and corneal edema, so I.O.P has to be maintained at a normal range.

---

*   **Ocular manifestations in AIDS**

Occurs in about 75% of patients.

1.   **Retinal microvasculopathy**

   *   Superficial & **deep** retinal hemorrhages occur in 15-40% cases,

   *   Multiple cotton wool spots occur in 50% cases.

   *   Microaneurysms & telagiectasia may also be seen rarely

2.   **Usual ocular infections :**

   *   Herpes zoster ophthalmicus

   *   Herpes simplex infections

   *   Toxoplasmosis (Chorioretinitis)

   *   Ocular tuberculosis, syphilis & fungal corneal ulcers

3.   **Opportunisitc infections**

   *   CMV retinitis

   *   Candida endophthalmits

   *   Cryptococcal infections

   *   Pneumocystis carini

   *   Choroiditis

4. **Unusual neoplasms :**

    *   Kaposi's sarcoma of eye lids & conjunctiva

    *   Burkitt's lymphoma of the orbit

5. **Neuro-ophthalmic lesion :** isolated or multiple cranial nerve palsies resulting in paralysis of eyelids, extra ocular muscles, loss of sensory supply to the eye & optic nerve.

    *   The most common abnormal findings on funduscopic examination are cotton-wool spots.

Corneal Vascularisation : Causes

Superficial

*   Superficial corneal ulcer

*   Contact lens user

*   Trachoma

*   Rosacea keratitis

*   Phlyctenulcar keratoconjuctivitis

Deep

*   Intestitial keratitis

*   Deep corneal ulcer

*   Chemical burns

*   Sclerosing keratitis

*   Disciform keratitis (occur in Herpes simplex keratitis

Grafts : There is a direct relationship b/w corneal neovascularisation & the severity of the allograft reaction.

Soft contact lens in particular are prone to producing superficial corneal neovascularisation. This is typically most prominent near the superior limbus.

*   **Hard exudates** are small, discrete, waxy looking with crenated margin whereas **soft exudates** have fluffy, indistinct margin.

* **Causes of Exudate**

Soft exudates	Hard exudates
Cotton wool spots spear as which fluffy spots with indistinct margins. Seen in.	Small discrete yellowish waxy areas with crenated margins. Seen in :
- Hypertensive retinpathy	- Diabetic retinopathy
- Toxaemic retinopathy of pregnancy	- Hypertensiive retinopathy
- Diabetic retinopathy	- Coat's disease
- Anemia	- Circinate retinopathy
- Collagen vascular disease like DLE, PAN, Scleroderma	

Aquaporins

* Aquaporins are a family of intrinsic membrane proteins that form pores or channels of water through cellular membranes in the presence of osmotic or hydrostatic radients (that allow transport of water)

* All molecules contain water channels that allow transport of water while some also contain channels for glycerol and may thus have limited permeability to glycerol.

Name	Water channels	Glycerol permeability	Mercury sensitivity	Localization
AQP0 (MIP)	+	+	+	Eye lens
AQP1 (CHIP28)	+	-	+	Erythrocytes, prox. tubules, eye brain, lung, blood vessels, inner ear, skeletal-heart, smooth muscles.
AQP2 (WCH-CD)	+	-	+	Collecting duct, endolymphatic sac
AQP3 (GLIP)	+	+	+	Collecting duct, conjunctiva, endolymphatic sac
AQP4 (MIWC)	+	-	+	Brain, lung, collecting duct eye, endolymphatic sac
AQP5	+	-	+	Lacrimal gland
AQP6 (hKID, AQP2L)	+	+	+	Kidney
AQP7	+	+	+	Sperm
AQP8	+	-	+	Sperm
AQP9	+	+	+	Adipose tissue

EMBRYOLOGY

THE DERIVATION OF OCULAR STRUCTURES FROM EMBRYONIC TISSUES

Surface ectoderm gives rise to :

* The lens
* The epithelium of the cornea.
* The epithelium of the conjunctiva and the lacrimal gland.
* The epithelium of the lids and its derivatives, the cilia, the meibomian glands, and the glands of Moll and Zeiss.
* The epithelial lining of the lacrimal passages.

Neural ectoderm gives rise to

* The retina (with its pigment epithelium).
* The epithelium covering the ciliary processes.
* The pigment epithelium covering the posterior surface of the iris.
* The sphincter and dilator pupillar muscles.
* The optic nerve (neuroglial, nervous elements and leptomeninges).
* Part of the vitreous body.

Surface and neural ectoderm gives rise to :

* Part of the vitreous and the suspensory ligament of the lens.
* Associated paraxial mesoderm gives to the blood vessels that persist (i.e. the choroidal, the central artery of the retina, the ciliary vessels and other vessels of the orbit) as well as the hyaloid artery, the vasa hyalodea propria, and the vessels of the vascular tunic of the lens that disappear before birth.
* The sclera
* The dural sheath of the optic nerve.

* The ciliary muscle

* The substantia propria of the cornea and the endothelium of its posterior surface.

* The stroma of the iris.

* The extrinsic muscles of the eye.

* The fat, ligaments, and other connective tissue structures in the orbit.

* The upper and inner walls of the orbit.

* The connective tissue of the upper lid.

Viseral mesoderm (maxillary process) below the eye gives rise to :

* The lower and outer walls of the orbit; the structures lying behind and below the eye (i.e. the alisphenoid and malar bones, and the orbital plate of the superior maxilla).

* The connective tissue of the lower lid.

SUMMARY OF THE CHRONOLOGY OF THE DEVELOPMENT OF THE EYES

PRE-EMBRYONIC PERIOD (Fertilization to end of third week)

* Formation of the principal germinal layers.

* Formation of neural plate and neural groove.

EMBRYONIC PERIOD (Beginning of 4th to End of 8th Week)

* Formation of the somites

* **25 days (14 somites, 2.6 mm)**

    — Appearance of the optic pits

* **26 to 28 days (19-25 somites, 3.2 mm)**

    — Evagination of optic vesicles.

    — Beginning formation of lens placode.

    — Condensation of mesoderm determining extraocular muscles.

* **5th week (3,4-8 mm)**

    — 4 to 4.2 mm

    Full development of primary optic vesicle.

    Earliest appearance of the primitive and marginal zones of the presumptive retina.

— **4.5 to 5 mm**

Beginning of invagination of optic vesicle of form optic cup.

Continued development of the retina with cellular differentiation.

Formation of the lens pit.

Ophthalmic artery emerges from internal carotid.

— **5.5 to 6 mm**

Rapid development of optic cup and development of embryonic fissure.

Hyaloid artery emerges from the primitive dorsal ophthalmic artery.

— **7 mm**

Optic vesicle fully invaginated and the embryonic fissure is open throughout its whole length.

Lens pit has developed into a closed vesicle in contact with the surfae ectoderm.

Hyaloid artery enters posterior embryonic fissure and reaches posterior pole of lens vesicle.

6th week (8-15 mm)

— **8 to 9 mm**

Continued differentiation of retina into cellular and marginal zones

Lens vesicle has become hollow sphere detached from the ectoderm

Hyaloid artery takes part in the formation of the posterior part of the tunica vasculosa lentis.

— **11 to 12 mm**

Beginning oo closure of embryonic cleft in its midportion.

Second stage of retinal differentiation with formation of primitive inner nuclear layer.

Formation of lens fibers from posterior cells of lens vesicle.

Mesodermal cells determining corneal endothelium begin growth as single layer under the surface epithelium.

— **13 to 14 mm**

Almost complete closure of embryonic fissure except at anterior and posterior extents.

Optic nerve fibers travelling proximally into optic nerve.

Cavity of lens vesicle much reduced and lens capsule completely formed.

Beginning development of secondary vitreous.

Choriocepillaries is complete.

Double layer of cells at the surface ectoderm forms the corneal epithelium.

Orbital mesoderm begins to differentiate into extraocular muscles.

7th week (15-22 mm)

— **15 to 16 mm**

Distal end of embryonic fissure completely closed.

Differentiation of inner and outer neuroblastic layers of retina effected by appearance of transient fiber layer of Chievitz at posterior pole.

Cavity of lens vesicle is obliterated.

Rudiments of lids have developed into definite folds and the fibers of the orbicularis oculi muscle begin to surround the eye.

17 to 18 mm

Retina continues to thicken and differentiate, reaching **0.175 mm**

Mesoderm determining future iris stroma takes shape and the scleral condensation becomes evident.

Formation of anterior portion of tunica vasculosa lentis.

— **20 to 21 mm**

Proximal remnant of embryonic fissure closed.

Retianl development proceeds to reach **0.19 mm** thickness.

Beginning of nerve fiber crossing to form optic chiasm.

Separation of corneal epithelial endothelium by acellular layer.

Nuclei of primary lens fibers disappear.

Tunica vasculosa lentis is completed and the vasa hyaloidea propria have appeared.

Lid fold gradually cover the eyes and the canaliculi are present.

8th week (22-30 mm)

— Retinal differentiation is proceeding rapidly

— Optic chiasm is fully formed

— Penetration of acellular layer of cornea by mesoderm to form the corneal stroma.

— Pupillary membrane is completely formed.

— Beginnings of anterior chamber can be discerned.

— Secondary lens fibers forming.

— Periocular mesodermal condensation determing the sclera has reached the equator.

— Lacrimal gland anlarge present.

— Further differentiation of mesodermal condensation determining the extracular muscles with evidence of fibrillae.

— All the ocular motor nerves have reached the extraocular muscles.

FETAL PERIOD (Beginning of 3rd Month to Birth)

* **9th week (30-40 mm)**

— Globe has reached **1 mm** in diameter.

— Ciliary body begins to appear.

— Hyaloid system is reaching maximal development.

— Secondary vitreous is fully evident.

— Y-sutures are now apparent in the embryonic nucleus of the lens

— Muscular fibers are evident in the mesoderm which forms the extra-ocular muscles.

* **10th week (40-50 mm)**

— The ciliary body is progressively formed.

— The ciliary musculature is forming and the zonule makes its appearance.

— Bowman's membrane is forming.

— Tenon's capsule begins to form in the equatorial region.

— Fibers of the orbicularis oculi are forming.

— Membranous bone is forming in the orbital walls.

— At the end of this period the optic tracts have formed.

* **11th week (50-60 mm)**
  — Macular area of the retina begins to differentiate.
  — Differentiation of the occipital cortex occurs.
  — The hyaloid system is maximally developed.
  — Rectus muscles are well differentiated and the levator separates from the superior rectus.

* **12th week (60-70 mm)**
  — Rudimentary rods and cones are forming in the retina.
  — Iris formation is occurring and the sphincter o fthe pupil appears.
  — The limbus is well demarcated and the canal of Schlemm emerges
  — Hyaloid system begins to atrophy.
  — Glial framework of the optic nerve begins to differentiate.
  — In the lids the enlarge of the tarsus is recognizable and the orbicularis is well developed.

* **4th month (70-110 mm)**
  — Globe increases in diameter from 3 to 7 mm.
  — Vascularization of the internal layers of the retina has begun.
  — Ciliary processes are fully formed and the middle layer of the choroid appears.
  — Posterior and lateral portions of the tunica vasculosa lentis regress.
  — The secondary vitreous develops considerably.
  — Lashes and glands of the lids appear and the plica is well formed.
  — Tenon's capsule is fully formed.
  — Orbital walls are well developed.

* **5th month (110-150 mm)**
  — Differentiation of the retina is progressive and the transient layer of Chievitz is obliterated except at the macula.
  — Myelination in the geniculate body is evident.
  — All layers of the choroid are now visible and melanoblasts appear in its external portion.
  — Fibers of the zonule run from the ciliary epithelium to the lens.
  — The iris is fully developed.
  — The extraocular muscles have differentiated their tendinous in sertions.
  — The dural sheath of the optic nerve can be distinguished.

* **6th month (150-200 mm)**

  — Foveolar depression is appearing in the macula.

  — The glial tissue of **Bergmeister's papilla** reaches its highest stage of development.

  — The dilator muscle of the pupil begins to form.

  — The sphincter muscle of the pupil is fully differentiated.

  — Descemet's membrane has appeared and the anterior chamber angle is forming peripherally.

* **7th month (200-230 mm)**

  — Diameter of the globe is 10 to 14 mm.

  — Rod cells are differentiated in the retina.

  — The fovea becomes obvious.

  — Myelination of the optic nerve fibers reaches the chiasm.

  — Bergmeister's papilla begins to atrophy.

  — The lacrimal canaliculi have opened onto the lid margins and the tarsus is well formed in the upper lids.

* **8th month (230-265 mm)**

  — All layers of the retina are extensively developed throughout.

  — Retinal vessels have reached the ora.

  — The fetal nucleus of the lens is complete.

  — The hyaloid system is rapidly disappearing.

  — The circulation of the anterior segment of the globe is complete.

  — The lids are separating throughout their length.

* **9th month (265-300 mm)**

  — Diameter of the globe increases to 16 to 17 mm.

  — Excepting the central area, the general structure of the retina is now complete.

  — Fibers of the infantile nucleus of the lens begin to appear.

  — The pupillary membrane and the hyaloid vessels have disappeared.

  — Begin formation of the physiologic cup of the disc.

* **At term**

— Apart from the fovea the retina is fully differentiated.

— Myelination of optic nerve fibers has reaches the lamina cribrosa.

— Coiled remnants of the haloid artery, attached anteriorly to the posterior lens capsule float freely in Cloquet's canal.

— The lacrimal gland is still undeveloped and tears are not secreted.

— The nasolacrimal passages have reached the nasal fossa but frequently are still separated from the inferior meatus by a membrane.

POSTNATAL PERIOD

Macula

Has lagged behing the rest of the retina and considerable changes occur after birth: differentiation of all layers proceeds during the first 4 months, at the end of which period the characteristic foveal reflex is present on ophthalmoscopy.

Fundus

Still lacks the pigmentation of the adult and the choroidal vessels are distinctly visible : "*salt and pepper*" appearance is due to the readily visible RPE : at the end of **6 months** the general picture approaches that of the adult fundus.

Lamina Cribrosa

Not fully developed until several months of age.

Upper Visual Pathways

Myelination proceeds from occipital cortex downward and is not complete until the end of the fourth month.

Visual reflex

Fixation Reflex

Present at birth weekly developed

Eye movement

Initially irregular and not conjugate but by 5 to 6 weeks the eyes can follow a light over a considerable range, pursuit of small objects occurs at about 3 months and transition from reflex to conscious fixation becomes apparent but conjugate fixation is not accurate until about 6 months, when convergence is established; corrective fusion reflexes are fully functional towards the end of the first year.

Blinking Reflex

Appears at about the 7th or 8th weeks

Uveal Tract

Undergoes considerable alteration after birth especially at the ciliary body; the dilator of the pupil is poorly developed and does not reach adult proportions until about the 5th year; the iris stromal pigment develops after birth in white races so that this tissue is initially light blue in color for some time.

Anterior Chamber Angle

Initially filled with uveal trabeculae but assumes adult configuration by **2 to 4 years of age.**

Cornea

Alternations occurs in the stroma and epithelium with decrease of stromal cellular elements and increase in fibrous elements while the epithelium grows from four layers of cells to five and six layers. The cornea also acquites a greater curvature from the initially flat appearance at birth but does not greatly increases in diameter.

Lens

Although, the infantile nucleus is present at birth it grows by accumulation of few fibers up to the age of puberty; after the continued accretion of new fibers forms of cortex; the lens capsule increass in thickness especially anteriorly; the hyaloid remnants at the posterior capsule gradually atrophy through childhood with variable trace remaining throughout life.

Anterior chamber

Initially deep but gradually shallows as the lens increases in A-P diameter.

Orbit

Undergoes considerable alteration in shape and grows progressively until puberty at which time it approximates adult size and shape.

Lacrimal Gland

Does not develop fully until 3 or 4 years of age and since the accessory lacrimal glands are few in number initially, there is little or no tearing for some weeks. Canalization of the lacrimal passages is delayed for several weeks to months and there may be a membrane obstructing the opening at the anferior meatus for a similar length of time.

CONJUNCTIVA

DIFFERENTIAL DIAGNOSIS BETWEEN FOLLICULAR CONJUNCTIVITIS, VERNAL CONJUNCTIVITIS AND TRACHOMA

		Follicular Conjunctivitis	*Vernal Conjunctivitis*	*Trachoma Stages I & II*
1.	Seasonal variation	Nil	Present	Nil
2.	Symptoms	Irritation with watering	Marked itching	Irritation with watering
3.	Follicles	Arranged in rows, never on pliac.	No follicles	Irregular arrangement, may appear on the plica.
4.	Papillae	None	Flat papillae cobble-stone	Fine papillae producing velvety appearance
5.	Conjunctival discharge	Slight discharge —mucoid or than muco-purulent	Ropy discharge	Watery, mucoid discharge
6.	Pannus	None	None	Always present
7.	Corneal involvement	None	Sometimes an opacity, like arcus seniles	Corneal ulcers, followed by opacities.

CLASSIFICATION : MacCallan first identified the value of a simple classification of *trachoma* for descriptive and therapeutic purposes.

Stage 1	Lymphoid follicles and subepithelial lymphoid infiltration. The follicles are hard, small and immature.
Stage 2(a)	In addition to a papillary response, mature follicles appear in the upper palpebral conjunctiva.
tage 2(b)	The papillary response becomes predominant, so that deep conjunctival vessels in the tarsal plate become obscured.
Stage 3	Follicles are present with early cicatrisation.
Stage 4	Follicles have disappeared, but cicatrisation is noted. The disease is inactive.
	The *WHO classification* records the presence or papillae (P) or follicles (F) and grades activity as mild, moderate or severe.
PO	Normal conjunctiva
P1 (mild)	Papillae are present, but the deep conjunctival vessels are not obscured.
P2 (moderate)	In addition to the presence of papillae, the conjunctive of upper tarsal plate is infiltration, so that the deep vessels are not visible.
P3 (severe)	Papillary response is marked and there is diffuse conjunctival infiltration and thickening the conjunctiva is opaque, distinguishing the deep vessels completely.
	The presence of follicles is described according to a series of zones. *Zone I* being near the upper margin of the tarsal plate. *Zone 2* being intermediate and *Zone 3* being the lowest and adjacent to the middle third of the lid margin.
FO	Normal conjunctiva without any follicles.
F1	Follicles are present, but not more than five in zones 1 and 2.
F2	More than five follicles in zones 1 and 2 but less than five in zone 3.
F3	Five or more follicles in each of the three zones.

THE RED EYE

	Conjunctivitis	Anterior uveitis	Acute glaucoma
Symptoms			
Pain	Minor-gritty or foreign	Present	Severe ocular pain and unilateral, frontal head-ache
Discharge	Present with sticki-ness in morning	Absent	Absent
Vision	Unaffacted	Blurred	Blurred-rainbow haloes around lights
Signs			
Hyperaemia	Superficial and diffuse most marked in fornices	Limbal	Diffuse and intense
Discharge	Mucoid, mucopuru-lent, or watery	Nil	Nil
Pre-auricular lymphnode	Palpable	Impalpable	Impalpable
Cornea	Clear	Clear-but KP visible with slit lamp	Oedematous
Intraocular pressure	Normal	Occasionally elevated	High

CORNEA

HYPERPLASTIC CORNEAL NERVES (Overgrowth of Corneal Nerves upto Twenty Times The Normal Number).

Non-specific changes may occur in association with the following.

1. Deep filiform dystrophy of Maeder and Danis
2. Herpes simplex
3. Herpes zoster
4. Neurofibromatosis (von Recklinghausen syndrome)
5. Neuroparalytic keratitis
6. Normal eyes at advanced age
7. Ocular pemphigus foliaceus (Cazenave disease)
8. Opaque corneal grafts
9. Phthisis bulbi
10. Posterior polymorphous dystrophy

Increased Visibility of Corneal Nerves

1. "Colloidin" skin syndrome (bullous ichthyosiform erythroderma)
2. Congenital
3. Ectodermal dysplasia (Rothmund syndrome)
4. Fuchs of dystrophy
5. Ichthyosis
6. Idiopathic
7. Keratoconus
8. Leprosy (Hansen disease)
9. Neurofibromatosis (von Recklinghausen syndrome)

MICROCORNEA (Cornea having a diameter of less than 10mm)

1. Associated ocular findings
    A. Aniridia and subluxated lenses
    B. Autosomal dominant cataract and myopia
    C. Autosomal dominant cataract, nystagmus and glaucoma
    D. Axenfeld syndrome (posterior embryotoxon)
    E. Colobomatous macrophthalmia
    F. Congenital glaucoma
    G. Corectopia and macular hypoplasia
    H. Hyperopia
    I. Meckel syndrome
    J. Nonophthalmos
    K. Narrow-angle glaucoma
    L. Sclerocornea
2. Aberfeld syndrome (congenital blepharophimosis associated with generalized myopathy).
3. Autosomal recessive or dominant trait.
4. Carpenter syndrome (acrocephalopolysyndactyly II).
5. Chromosome 18 partial deletion (long-arm) syndrome.
6. Ehlers-Danlos syndrome (fibrodysplasia elastica generalisata).
7. Gansslen syndrome.
8. Hallermann-Streff syndrome (dyscephalia mandibulo-oculo-facialis)
9. Hemifacial microsomia syndrome.
10. Hutchinson-Gilford syndrome (Progeria).
11. Laurence-Moon-Biedle syndrome (retinitis pigmentosa-polydactyly-adiposo-genital syndrome).
12. Lenz microphthalmia syndrome.
13. Little syndrome (nail patella syndrome).
14. Locally associated with hyperopia, narrow-angle glaucoma, congenital glaucoma, or sclerocornea.
15. Marchesani syndrome (mesodermal dysmorphodystrophy).
16. Marfan's syndrome (dolichostenomelia-arachnodactyly-hyperchondroplasia-dystrophica mesodermalis congenita).

17. Meckel syndrome (dysencephalia splanchnocystic syndrome).

18. Meyer-Schnickerath-Weyers syndrome (oculodentiodigital dysplasia).

19. Rieger syndrome (hypodontia and iris dysgenesis).

20. Rubella syndrome.

21. Sabin-Feldman syndrome.

22. Schwartz syndrome (glaucoma associated with retinal detachment).

23. Trisomy 13-15 (D trisomy).

24. Waardenberg syndrome (interoculoiridodermatoauditive dysplasia).

MEGALOCORNEA (Cornea having a horizontal diameter of more than 14 mm)

1. Aarskog syndrome (facial digital genital syndrome).

2. Autosomal dominant or recessive trait.

3. Congenital glaucoma (rare).

4. Marchesani syndrome (brachymorphy with spherophakia).

5. Marfan syndrome (dystrophia mesodermalis congenita).

6. Mucopolysaccharidosis I-S (Scheie syndrome).

7. Oculocerebrorenal syndrome (Lowe syndrome).

8. Oculodental syndrome (micrognathia-glossoptosis syndrome).

9. Osteogenesis imperfecta (van der Hoeve syndrome).

10. Pierre-Robin syndrome (micrognathia-glossoptosis syndrome).

11. Posterior embryotoxon.

12. Rieger syndrome (hypodontia and iris syndrome).

13. Rubella syndrome (Gregg syndrome).

14. Sex-linked recessive trait.

15. Sturge-Weber syndrome (meningocutaneous syndrome).

KERATOCONUS (Conical Cornea (Noninflammatory Ectasia of Cornea in its axial part with considerable visual impairment because of development of a high degree of irregular myopic astigmatism)

Keratoconus may be associated with :

1. Acute hydrops of the cornea.
2. Aniridia.
3. Apert syndrome (acrodysplasia).
4. Asthma, hay fever.
5. Atopic dermatitis, keratosis plantaris, and palmaris.
6. Blue sclerotics, including van der Hoeve syndrome (osteogenesis imperfecta).
7. Chandler syndrome (iridocorneal endothelial syndrome).
8. Contact lens wear.
9. Ehlers-Danlos syndrome (fibrodysplasia elastica generalisata).
10. Gronblad-Strandberg syndrome (pseudoxanthoma elasticum).
11. Hereditary history.
12. Hyperextensible joints and mitral valve prolapse.
13. Infantile tapetoretinal degeneration of Leber.
14. Laurence-Moon-Biedl syndrome (retinitis polydactyly-adiposogenital syndrome).
15. Little syndrome (nail-patella syndrome).
16. Lymphogranuloma venereum.
17. Marfan syndrome (hypoplastic form of dystrophia mesodermalis congenita).
18. Monogolism (Down syndrome).
19. Neurodermatitis.
20. Neurofibromatosis (von Recklinghausen syndrome)
21. Noonan syndrome (male Turner syndrome).
22. Pellucid marginal corneal degeneration.
23. Retinal disinsertion corneal degeneration.
24. Retinitis pigmentosa.
25. Retrolental fibroplasia.
26. Trauma, such as birth injury or contussion.
27. Vernal catarrh.

CORNEAL PIGMENTATON

Type of pigment	Cause	Location
Iron	Keratoconus (**Fleischer's ring**)	Epithelium
	Old age (**Hudson stapli line**)	Epithelium
	Pterygium (**Stocker's line**)	Epithelium
	Filtering bleb(**Ferry's line**)	Epithelium
	Hyphaema-blood staining	Mainly stroma
	Siderosis	Mainly stroma
Silver	Argyrosis	Stroma & Descemet's
Gold	Chrysiasis	Mainly epithelium
Copper	Wilson's disease (**Kayser-Fleischer ring**)	Descemet's
Melanin	Pigment dispersion syndrome (Krukenberg's spindle)	Endothelium

SCLERA

BLUE SCLERA (Localized or generalized blue coloration of Sclera because of thinness and loss of water content allowing underlying dark choroid to be seen)

1. Albright hereditary osteodystrophy (pseudohypoparathyroidism).
2. Bloch-Sulzberger syndrome (incontinentia pigmenti).
3. Brittle cornea syndrome (blue sclera syndrome)—recessive.
4. Corneal encroachment into sclera.
5. Crouzon disease (craniofacial dysostosis).
6. de Lange syndrome (congenital muscular hypertrophy—cerebral syndrome).
7. Ehler-Danlos syndrome (fibrodysplasia elastica generalisata)
8. Folling syndrome (phenylketonuria).
9. Goltz syndrome (focal dermal hypoplasia syndrome).
10. Hallerman-Streiff syndrome (dyscephalia mandibulo-oculo-facial syndrome).
11. Hypophosphatasia (phosphoethanolaminuria).
12. Lowe syndrome (oculocerebrorenal syndrome).
13. Marfan syndrome (dystrophia mesodermalis congenita).
14. Osteogenesis imperfecta (van der Hoeve syndrome).
15. Paget syndrome (osteitis deformans).
16. Pierre-Robin syndrome (micrognathia-glossoptosis syndrome)
17. Pycnodysostosis
18. Relapsing polychondritis
19. Staphyloma
20. Turner 's syndrome (gonadal dysgenesis)
21. Werner syndrome (progeria of adults)

ANTERIOR CHAMBER OF THE EYE

NARROW ANTERIOR CHAMBER ANGLE
(May be capable of angle closure glaucoma)

1. Normal variation
2. Predisposition to angle closure
3. Anterior dislocation of the lens
4. Hyperope
5. Spherophakia and microcornea
6. Postoperative intraocular operation with leaking wound.
7. Choroidal detachment
8. Pupillary block
9. Loss of aqueous from perforating ulcer, corneal wound, or staphyloma.
10. Intumescent senile cataract
11. Traumatic cataract that fluffs- up
12. Primary hyperplastic, primary vitreous
13. Peripheral anterior synechiae
14. Posterior entrapment of aqueous humor (malignant glaucoma of ciliary-block glaucoma).
15. Drugs, including; acetazolamide, acetylcholine, alpha-chymotrypsin, demecarium, dichlorphenamide, echothiophate, edrophonium, ethoxzolamide, isoflurophate, methazolamide, neostigmine, physostigmine, pilocarpine, sulfacetamide, sulfachlorpyridazine, sulfadiazine, sulfadimethoxine, sulfamerazine, sulfameter, sulfamethizole, sulfamethoxazole, sulfamethoxypyridazine, sulfanilamide, sulfaphenazole, sulfisoxazole

PHYSIOLOGIC MYDRIASIS (Dilated Pupil)
(*Usually greater than 5mm*)

A. Larger pupils in women than in men.

B. Larger pupils in myopes than in hypermetropes.

C. Larger pupils in blue irides than in brown irides.

D. Larger pupils in adolescents and middle-aged persons than in very young or old persons.

E. Voluntary dilatation (rare) by respiratory suspension and acceleration of heart beat.

F. Surprise, fear, pain, strong emotion, or vestibular stimulation.

G. General anaesthesia of stages I, II, and IV.

H. Autosensory pupillary reflex—stimulation of middle ear.

I. Auditory pupillary reflex—tuning fork adjacent to ear.

J. Vestibular pupillary reflex — stimulation of labyrinth by heat, cold, or rotation.

K. Vagotonic pupillary reflex—stimulation on deep inspiration.

FIXED, DILATED PUPIL

1. *Midbrain damage*—vascular accidents, tumors, degenerative and infectious disease.

    A. Dorsal (Edinger-Westphal nucleus and its connections)—Rare involves both pupils, pupillary near vision reaction often retained, and often associated with supranuclear vertical gaze palsy.

    B. Ventral (fascicular part of third nerve)—Associated with other neurologic deficits, such as Nothangel syndrome, Benedikt syndrome, Weber syndrome to spare the extraocular components of the third nerve.

2. *Damage to the third nerve* (from interpeduncular fossa to ciliary ganglion).

    A. Basal aneurysms

    B. Supratentorial space—Occupying masses, causing displacement of the brain stem or transtentorial herniation of the uncus; stuporous or comatose.

3. *Damage to the ciliary ganglion* or short ciliary nerves—results in Adie tonic pupil

4. *Damage to the iris*

   A. Degenerative or inflammatory disease of the iris.

   B. Posterior synechiae.

   C. Acute rise of intraocular pressure (hypoxia or sphincter damage).

   D. Blunt injury to the globe with sphincter damage (traumatic iridoplegia).

   E. Pharmacologic blockade by atropinic substances.

5. *Total blindness,* including cortical blindness

PHYSIOLOGIC MIOSIS (Small Pupil) (*Usally less than 2mm*)

A. Smaller pupil in men than in women.

B. Smaller pupil in hypermetropes than in myopes.

C. Smaller pupil in brown irides than in blue irides.

D. Smaller pupil in very young or old persons than in adolescents and middle-aged persons.

E. Sleep, fatigue, coma.

F. Stage III anesthesia

G. Orbicularis reflex

   Reader paratrigeminal syndrome—ipsilateral miosis and pain—may by associated with third-nerve paralysis or corneal anesthesia

   A. Idiopathic   B. Migraine

   C. Meningioma   D. Post-trauma

   E. Extracranial aneurysm of internal carotid

ARGYLL ROBERTSON PUPIL—small and irregular; reacts better to accommodation than to light

A. Syphilis (acquired lues).

B. Diabetes mellitus (Willis disease).

C. Chronic alcoholism

D. Different kinds of encephalitis.

E. Multiple sclerosis (disseminated sclerosis).

F. Senile and degenerative diseases of the central nervous system.

G. Midbrain tumors, such as pinealomas and craniopharyngioma.

H. Friedreich ataxia.

I. Malaria.

J. Syringomyelia.

K. Carbon disulfide poisoning.

L. Herpes zoster, usually mydriasis.

M. Pressure on third cranial nerve trunk by cerebral aneurysm.

N. Trauma to skull or orbit.

O. Aberrant regeneration of the third nerve.

PERSISTENT PUPILLARY MEMBRANE

*   = Most important

1. Fetal iritis

2. Hereditary

3. Physiologic

* 4. Use of oxygen therapy in premature nursery

DECENTERED PUPILLARY LIGHT REFLEX

1. Positive angle kappa—Pseudoexotropia.

2. Negative angle kappa—Pseudoesotropia.

3. Eccentric fixation—Deep unilateral amblyopia.

4. Ectopic macula—Macular displacement by retinal scarring or strands, such as retrolental fibroplasia.

5. Ectopic pupil.

UVEAL TRACT

RUBEOSIS IRIDIS (Neovascularization [Newly Formed Blood Vessles] on iris)

* = Most important

1. Proximal vascular disease

   A. Aortic arch syndrome (pulseless disease; Takayasu syndrome).

   B. Carotid-cavernous fistula carotid artery syndrome).

   C. Carotid ligation

   D. Carotid occlusive disease

   E. Cranial arteritis syndrome (giant-cell arteritis).

2. Ocular vascular disease

   A. Central retinal artery thrombosis

   B. Central retinal vein thrombosis

   C. Long posterior ciliary artery occlusion

   D. Reversed flow through the ophthalmic artery

3. Retinal diseases

   A. Coats disease (retinal telangiectasia)

   B. Diabetes mellitus

   C. Eales disease (periphlebitis)

   D. Glaucoma, chronic

   E. Melanoma of choroid

   F. Norrie disease (oligophrenia-microphthalmos syndrome)

   G. Persistent hyperplastic primary vitreous

   H. Retinal detachment

    I. Retinal hemangioma

    J. Retinoblastoma

    K. Retrolental fibroplasia

    L. Sickle cell disease (Herrick syndrome)

4. Iris tumors

    A. Hemangioma

    B. Melanoma

    C. Metastatic carcinoma

5. Postinflammatory

    A. Argon laser coreoplasty

    B. Exfoliation syndrome

    C. Fibrinoid syndrome

    D. Fungal endophthalmitis

    E. Iris neovascularization with pseudoexfoliation

    F. Radiation

    G. Retinal detachment operation

    H. Uveitis, chronic

6. Vascular tuffs at the pupillary margin

    A. Cataract

    B. Diabetes mellitus

    C. Myotonic dystrophy syndrome (myotonia atrophica syndrome)

    D. Ocular hypotony

    E. Respiratory failure

HYPEREMIA OF IRIS
(Dilatation of Pre-existing Vessels of Iris)

1. Corneal ulcer
2. Foreign body on the cornea
3. Injury, intraocular
4. Iridocyclitis
5. Iritis
6. Scleritis
7. Uveitis

IRIDODONESIS (tremulousness)

1. Aphakia following cataract extraction
2. Dislocation of the lens
3. Hydrophthalmos or buphthalmos
4. Hypermature senile cataract

CONDITIONS SIMULATING ANTERIOR UVEITIS OR IRITIS

1. Brushfield spots
2. Fuchs syndrome (II) Stevens-Johnson syndrome).
3. Hereditary deep dystrophy of cornea
4. Hyalinized keratitic precipitate
5. Iridoschisis—splitting of iris
6. Juvenile xanthogranuloma of the iris (nevoxantho-endothelioma).
7. Malignant lymphomas or leukemia
8. Malignant melanoma
9. Metastatic tumor arising from the lungs, breast, gastrointestinal tract, thyroid, gland, prostate gland, kidney, or testicle.
10. Neurofibromas of the iris
11. Pigment floaters in the anterior chamber, especially after mydriasis.
12. Pseudoexfoliation of the lens capsule (glaucoma capsulare).
13. Reticulum cell sarcoma
14. Retinoblastoma
15. Scleroderma (progressive systemic sclerosis).
16. Siderosis bulbi

PSEUDOENDOPHTHALMITIS
(Conditions that simulate endophthalmitis)

1. Chemical reactions from irritating chemicals introduced into the anterior chamber.
2. Foreign material in the anterior chamber.
3. Metastatic carcinoma
4. Retained lenticular material
5. Severe postoperative iridocyclitis

INTRAOCULAR CALCIFICATIONS

1. Choroidal osteoma
2. Facial nevus of Jadassohn (linear sebaceous nevus syndrome).
3. Intraocular calcifications
   A. Congenital deformity
   B. Recurrent iritis and keratitis
   C. Retinal detachment
   D. Trauma (perforating, nonperforating, or surgical).
4. Intraocular sarcoma
5. Retinoblastoma
6. Retrolental fibroplasia
7. Sites of intraocular calcification
   A. Calcific emboli of retinal and ciliary arteries.
   B. Cyclitic membrane
   C. Lens
   D. Peripapillary choroid
   E. Posterior pole to ora serrata in region of choroid and pigment epithelium.
   F. Retina
   G. Vitreous

PHTHISIS BULBI (Degenerative shrinkage of Eyeball with hypotony)

1. Following cataract surgery, especially with rubella syndrome (German measles).
2. Panophthalmitis
3. Severe ocular injury with loss of tissue
4. Severe uveitis
5. Sympathetic ophthalmia
6. Tumor, such as retinoblastoma or malignant melanoma.

ANGIOID STREAKS (Ruptures of bruch membrane characterized Ophthalmoscopically by brownish lines surrounding the Disc and Radiating toward the Periphery)

1. Acromegaly
2. Cardiovascular disease with hypertension
3. Cooley anemia
4. Diffuse lipomatosis
5. Dwarfism
6. Epilepsy
7. Facial angiomatosis
8. Fibrodysplasia hyperelastica (Ehlers-Danlos syndrome).
9. Francois dyscephalic syndrome (Hallermann-Streff syndrome).
10. Lead poisoning
11. Ocular melanocytosis
12. Osteitis deformans (Paget's disease)
13. Pituitary tumor
14. Previous choroidal detachment
15. Pseudoxanthoma elasticum (Gronblad-Strandberg syndrome).
16. Senile (actinic) elastosis of the skin
17. Sickle cell disease (Herrick syndrome)
18. Thrombocytopenic purpura

LENS

IRIDESCENT CRYSTALLINE DEPOSITS IN LENS

1. Idiopathic
2. Hypothyroid (cretinism)
3. Hypocalcemia

    A. Postoperative—Removal of thyroid and accidental parathyroid removal.

    B. Idiopathic hypoparathyroidism.

    C. Pseudohypoparathyroidism (hypoparathyroid cretinism) or with hyper- phosphatemia (Albright disease).

    D. Pseudopseudohypoparathyroidism (brachymetacarpal dwarfism).

4. Myotonic dystrophy (Curschmann-Steinert syndrome).
5. Drugs, including carhenazine, chlorpromazine, chloroprothixene, colloidal silver, diazepam, diethazine, ethopropazine, fluphenazine, gold Au 198, gold sodium thiomalate, mercuric oxide, mesoridazine, methdilazine, methotrimeprazine, mild silver protein, perazine, pericyazine, perphenazine, phenylmercuric acetate, phenylmercuric nitrate, piperacetazine, prochlorperazine, promazine, promethazine, propiomazine, silver nitrate, silver protein, thiopropazate, thioridazine, thiothixene, trifluoperazine, triflupromazine, trimeprazine.
6. Cataract (coroaliform and aculeiform) usually autosomal dominant; sometimes recessive.

OIL DROPLET IN LENS

1. Anterior displacement of lens.
2. Galactosemia-transferase deficiency (von Reuss syndrome).
3. Lenticonus

LENTICONUS (Conical, lens surface protuberance) AND LENTIGLOBUS (Globular lens surface protuberance)

1. Anterior—rare and usually bilateral.

    A. Alport syndrome (hereditary nephritis).

    B. Spina bifida.

    C. Waardenburg syndrome (embryonic fixation syndrome).

2. Posterior—more common and often unilateral.

    A. May be associated with persistent hyperplastic primary vitreous.

    B. May be associated with remnants of hyloid artery.

    C. Lowe syndrome (oculocerebrorenal syndome).

    D. Trauma.

LENS ABSORPTION

1. Congenital rubella syndrome (German measles).

2. Hallerman-Streiff syndrome (dyscephalic mandibulo-oculo facial syndrome).

3. Surgical trauma as discission.

4. Trauma, blunt or penetrating.

MICROPHAKIA OR SPHEROPHAKIA (Small Lens or Highly Spherical Lens)

1. Achard syndrome (Marfan syndrome with dysostosis mandibulofacialis).

2. Alport syndrome (hereditary nephritis).

3. Familial anomaly

4. Homocystinuria syndrome

5. Hyperlysinemia

6. Lenticular myopia as recessive inheritance trait.

7. Little syndrome (hereditary osteo-orcychodysplasia)

8. Lowe syndrome (renal rickets).

9. Marchesani syndrome (brachymorphy with spherophakia).

10. Marfan syndrome (dolichostenomelia-arachnodactyly hyperchondroplasia dystrophica mesodermalis congenita).

11. Reticular dystrophy of the retinal pigment epithelium.

12. Rubella syndrome (Gregg syndrome).

13. Waardenburg syndrome (embryonic fixation syndrome)

DISEASES OF THE VITREOUS

PSEUDODETACHMENT OF VITREOUS (Conditions simulating detachment of Vitreous)

1. Enormous cavity in the vitreous body with a relatively thin posterior wall.

2. Membranous formations within the vitreous associated with uveitis and haemorrhage.

3. Outline of the ascending portion of cloquet canal just anterior to the disc.

ANTERIOR VITREOUS DETACHMENT
(Anterior Vitreous may be separated from Posterior Lens or Posterior Zonular Fibers)

1. Retrolenticular—usually caused by vitreous shrinkage
   - A. Trauma
   - B. Haemorrhage
   - C. Senescence
   - D. Inflammation
   - E. Retinal detachment
2. Retrozonular
   - A. Vitreous shrinkage
   - B. Ciliary body tumor
   - C. Blood
   - D. Exudate
3. Retrolenticular and retrozonular combined occurs with rupture of the hyaloideocapsular ligament.

POSTERIOR VITREOUS DETACHMENT

1. Complete posterior detachment
A. Simple detachment—occurs in young persons.

   (i) Exduate from chorioretinitic focus.

   (ii) Haemorrhage between the vitreous and the retina.

(iii) Retraction of the cortical vitreous caused by exudate within the vitreous.

(iv) Vitreous haemorrhage in a young individual with vitreous shrinking because of thrombosis of central retinal vein, retinitis proliferans, central serous retinopathy, or trauma.

B. Complete posterior detachment with collapse

   (i) Senescent changes are primary cause

   (ii) Uveitis

   (iii) Trauma

   (iv) Haemorrhage

   (v) Sodium hyaluronate

C. Funnel-shapped posterior detachment

   (i) Perforating injuries of globe

   (ii) Retinitis proliferans

   (iii) Massive vitreous detachment

D. Atypical complete posterior detachment—residual adherence of vitreous to a peripheral retinal area

   (i) Focus of chorioretinitis

   (ii) Following cataract extraction with loss of vitreous

   (iii) Following perforating wounds

2. Partial posterior detachment (unusual)

A. Superior detachment—primarily a senescent changes, generally forerunner of posterior vitreous detachment with collapse.

B. Partial posterior detachment (not infrequent)

   (i) Preretinal haemorrhage

   (ii) Retinitis proliferans

C. Partial lateral or partial inferior detachment

   (i) Focus of choroiditis

   (ii) Circumscribed retinal periphlebitis

   (iii) Intraocular foreign body

BEADS IN VITREOUS (Snowballs in Vitreous)

1. African eyeworm disease Iloiasis)
2. Amyloidosis (Lubarsch-Pick syndrome)
3. Bang disease (Brucellosis)
4. Behcet syndrome (Dermatostomato-ophthalmic syndrome)
5. Criswick-Schepens syndrome (familial exudative vitreoretinopathy)
6. Hemophilus influenzae
7. Irvine syndrome
8. Jacobsen-Brodwall syndrome
9. Japanese river fever (typhus)
10. Oculo-oto-ororenoerythropoietic disease
11. Pars planitis
12. Retinoblastoma
13. Sarcoid (Schaumann syndrome)
14. Severe uveitis
15. Toxic lens syndrome
16. Vogt-Koyanagi-Harada syndrome (uveitis-vitiligo-alopecia-poliosis syndrome)

VITREOUS LIQUEFACTION

1. Myopia
2. Peripheral uveitis
3. Retinitis pigmentosa
4. Spontaneous
5. Trauma
6. With aging
7. With vitreous traction as Wagener disease

GLAUCOMA

DIFFERENTIAL DIAGNOSIS BETWEEN BUPHTHALMOS AND MEGALOCORNEA

Buphthalmos	*Megalocornea*
1. Familial occurrence rare.	1. Familial occurrence common
2. Males to females = 5 : 3	2. Almost entirely in males
3. Unilateral in 35% of cases	3. Bilateral
4. Corneal opacities and ruptures in Descemet's membrane	4. No corneal opacities.
5. Visual impairment is marked	5. No visual impairment
6. Intra-ocular tension raised	6. No rise of tension
7. Gross abnormalities at the angle of the anterior chamber	7. No malformation at the angle
8. Cupping of the disc present.	8. No cupping of the disc.

LOW-TENSION GLAUCOMA OR PSEUDO-GLAUCOMA

This is a condition which is not glaucoma in the true sense. It occurs bilaterally in elderly perosn. There are cupping of the disc and visual field changes similar to those in chronic simple glaucoma. The angle of the anterior chamber is also wide. But the intra-ocular pressure remains either normal or subnormal. This pressure does not elevate during diurnal variations and also it cannot be raised by provocative tests. The cupping and the field changes are due to vascular insufficiency of the optic nerve-head and the optic nerve. Thus this condition should be best considered as ischaemic neuropathy of the optic nerve.

CHERRY RED SPOT IN MACULA
(Rule out macular Haemorrhage)

1. b-Galactoosidase deficiency (mucopolysaccharidosis 9 MPS) VII
2. Cardiac myxomas
3. Cryoglobulinemia
4. Hallevorden-Spartz disease (pigmentary degeneration of globus pallidus)
5. Hollenhorst syndrome (chorioretinal infarction syndrome)
6. Hurler syndrome (MPS I-H)
7. Hypertension (severe)
8. Intralesional chalazion corticosteroid injection
9. Macular retinal hole with surrounding detachment
10. Mucolipidosis-I (lipomucopolysaccharidosis)
11. Myotonic dystrophy syndromy (Curschmann-Steinert syndrome)
12. Occlusion of central retinal artery
13. Quinine toxicity
14. Sphingo-lipidoses

    A. Cherry-red spot myoclonus

    B. Farber syndrome (Farber lipogranulomatosis)

    C. Gangliosidosis (GMI—type 2 (juvenile gangliosidosis)

    D. Gaucher disease (glucocerebroside storage disease)

    E. Goldberg syndrome

    F. Infantile metachromatic leukodystrophy (van Bogaert-Nijssen disease)

    G. Niemann-Pick disease (essential lipoid histiocytosis)

    H. Sandoff disease (gangliosidosis GM2—type 2)

    I. Tay-Sachs disease (familial amaurotic idiocy)

15. Temporal arteries (Hutchinson—Horton Magrath-Brown syndrome)
16. Traumatic retinal edema (commotio retinae; Berlin edema)
17. Vogt-Spielmeyer cerebral degeneration (Batten-Mayou syndrome).

DISEASES OF THE RETINA

DIFFERENTIAL DIAGNOSIS BETWEEN PSEUDO-GLIOMA AND RETINOBLASTOMA

	Pseudoglioma	*Retinoblastoma*
1. Nature of the disease	1. Inflammatory in origin and it is the terminal phase of endophthalmitis	1. It is a neoplasm
2. Inflammatory	2. a) Ciliary flush b) Posterior synechia c) K. P.	2. Nil
3. Tension	3. Usually low or normal	3. High
4. Progress	4. Non-progressive	4. Progressive

LESION CONFUSED WITH RETINOBLASTOMA

1. Anomalous optic disc
2. Anterior dislocated lens with secondary glaucoma
3. Coats disease (retinal telangiectasia)
4. Coloboma of choroid and optic disc
5. Congenital corneal opacity
6. Congenital rubella syndrome (Gregg syndrome)
7. Cysts in a remnant of the hyaloid artery
8. Developmental retinal cyst
9. Glioma of the retina
10. Hematoma under retinal pigment epithelium

11. High myopia with advanced chorioretinal degeneration

12. Juvenile retinoschisis

13. Juvenile xanthogranuloma (nevoxanthoendothelioma)

14. Larval granulomatosis (Toxocara canis)

15. Medullation of nerve fiber layer

16. Metastatic endophthalmitis

17. Norrie disease (atrophia oculi congenita)

18. Oligodendrogliooma of the retina

19. Organization of intraocular haemorrhage

20. Persistent hyperplastic primary vitreous

21. Retinal detachment due to choroidal or vitreous haemorrhage

22. Retinal dysplasia (massive retinal fibrosis)

23. Retrolental fibroplasia

24. Retrolental membrane associated with Bloch-Sulzberger syndrome (incontinentia pigmenti)

25. Rhegmatogenous and falciform retinal detachment

26. Secondary glaucoma

27. Sex-linked microphthalmia

28. Tapetoretinal degeneration

29. Trisomy 13-15 (Patau syndrome)

30. Toxoplasmosis (ocular toxoplasmosis)

31. Traumatic chorioretinitis

32. Tumors other than retinoblastoma

33. Uveitis in secondary retinal detachment

34. *'White-with pressure'* sign.

LESIONS OF THE VISUAL PATHWAYS

1. *Lesions of the optic nerve*

   (a) Affection of the papillomacular bundle produces central scotoma.

   (b) Affection of temporal or nasal fibres of the nerve causes corresponding field defects, e.g. temporal lesion causes defect in the nasal field and vice versa.

   (c) Total lesion of the optic nerve causes total blindness due to optic atrophy.

2. *Lesions of the optic chiasma*

   Usual field defect is bitemporal hemianopia, i.e. loss of temporal field of vision in each eye, due to the affection of the crossed fibres from the nasal half of each retina.

   Binasal hemianopia, is extremely rare. It is produced by lesions on either side of the chiasma, so that the uncrossed fibres from the temporal half of each retina are affected. In both the conditions, there is partial optic atrophy.

3. *Lesions of the optic tract*

   The usual field defect is homonymous hemianopia, i.e. loss of nasal field of the same side and temporal field of the opposite side. Due to proximity of the crus cerebri and oculomotor nerves to the tracts, ocular palsies and hemiplegia may by associated with tract lesions. There is also partial optic atrophy.

   Right homonymous hemianopia causes difficulty in reading.

4. *Lesions of the lateral geniculate body*

   The field defect caused by this lesion is also homonymous hemianopia.

5. *Lesions of optic radiations.*

Lesion across the entire radiation produces homonymous hemianopic field defect. There is no optic atrophy and pupil reactions are normal.

A lesion in the upper or lower part of the radiation produces quadrantic hemianopia in which corresponding quadrants of each field are lost.

6. *Lesions of the visual cortex*

If the lesion is extensive as due to thrombosis of the calcarine artery, the field defect is homonymous hemianopia with sparing of the fixation area. But if only the areas above or below the calcarine fissure are affected, quadrantic hemianopia is produced.

PSEUDO-OPTIC NEURITIS
(Lesions that Mimic Optic Neuritis)

1. Central scotomas produced by expanding lesions of anterior and middle cranial fossa.

   A. Craniopharyngiomas

   B. Ectopic pinealomas

   C. Hodgkin disease

   D. Lymphomas

   E. Meningiomas

   F. Metastatic carcinomas

   G. Nasopharyngeal carcinomas

   H. Plasmacytoma

   I. Pituitary adenomas

2. Blurring of the disc from drusen or papilledema.

3. Ischemic optic neuropathy.

4. Retinal lesions that also exhibit metamorphosia, such as severe or angiospastic retinopathy.

5. Tumors of disc, such as metastatic carcinoma, gliomas, neurofibromas, hematomas, and meningiomas.

PSEUDOPAPILLEDEMA (May be mistaken for swelling of optic nerve)

1. Arteriovenous aneurysms (recemose aneurysms) of the retina (Wyburn-Mason syndrome).

2. Cervico-oculoacousticus syndrome.

3. Drusens of optic nerve

4. Epipapillary membrane and Bergmeister papilla.

5. High hyperopia or astigmatism.

6. Medullated nerve fibers (opaque nerve fibers).

7. Normal variant

8. Opacities or haziness of the media, especially nuclear sclerosis of the lens.

9. Optic neuritis or papillitis.

10. Tortuosity and anomalous early branching of the retinal vessels.

11. Tumors of disc, such as gliomas, meningiomas, neurinomas, neurofibromas, metastatic tumor, hematoma, and sarcoid.

PSEUDOESOTROPIA (Ocular appearance of esotropia when no manifest deviation of visual axis is present)

1. Abnormal shape of skull or abnormal thickness of skin surrounding the orbits.

2. Enophthalmos

3. Entropion

4. Hypotelorism with narrow interpupillary distance.

5. Lateral displacement of the concavity of the upper eyelid margin from the centre of the pupil.

6. Negative angle kappa—pupillary light reflex displaced temporarily.

7. Prominent epicanthal fold.

8. Telecanthus—The orbits are normally placed, but the medial canthi are far apart secondary to lateral displacement of the soft tissue.

PSEUDOEXOTROPIA (Ocular appearance of exotropia when no manifest deviation of visual axis is present)

1. Displaced macula (heterotropia of the macula).

2. Heterochromia when the lighter colored eye appears to diverge.

3. Hypertelorism with wide interpupillary distance.

4. Exophthalmos

5. Positive-angle kappa—pupillary light reflex displaced nasally.

6. Narrow lateral canthus

7. Wide palpebral fissure

PAINFUL OPHTHALMIPLEGIA
(Palsy of ocular muscles with pain)

1. Adenocarcinoma metastatic to the orbit.
2. Alternating exophthalmos with painful ophthalmoplegia.
3. Atypical facial neuralgia.
4. Cavernous sinus syndrome (Foix syndrome).
5. Collier sphenoidal palsy.
6. Diabetic ophthalmoplegia.
7. Intracavernous carotid aneurysm.
8. Nasopharyngeal tumor.
9. Ophthalmoplegic migraine.
10. Orbital abscess.
11. Orbital axex sphenoidal syndrome (Rollet syndrome).
12. Orbital myositis
13. Orbital periositis
14. Osteoperiostitis, anterior (orbital).
15. Osteoperiostitis, posterior (orbital).
16. Postherpetic neuralgia
17. Pseudotumor of orbit
18. Superior orbital fissure syndrome (Rochon-Duvigneaud syndrome, including superior orbital fissuritis).
19. Tic douloureux of the first trigeminal division.
20. Tolosa-Hunt syndrome (inflammatory lesion of cavernous sinus).

TRANSIENT OPHTHALMOPLEGIA (Extraocular muscle paralysis of short duration)

1. Following internal carotid artery ligation for treatment of intracavernous giant aneurysm.

2. Intrathecal chemotherapy and cranial irradiation.

3. Lethargic encephalitis.

4. Multiple sclerosis (disseminated sclerosis)—usually the lateral rectus.

5. Oculomotor nuclear complex infarction.

6. Recurrent oculomotor palsy.

7. Syphilis (acquired lues)

8. Tabes

9. Treatment of arteriovenous fistulas with Debrum balloon technique.

10. Wilson disease (hepatolenticular degeneration)

PSEUDOPTOSIS (Conditions simulating ptosis, but lid droop is not the result of levator malfunction, and process is usually corrected when the causative factors are cleared up or removed)

1. Globe displacement

   A. Anophthalmia including poorly fitting prosthesis.

   B. Enophthalmos such as that resulting from blow-out fracture of the floor of the orbit or atrophy of orbital fat.

   C. Microphthalmia

   D. Phthisis bulbi

   E. Hypotonia and inward collapse of eye.

   F. Cornea plana

   G. Hypotonia of that eye or hypertropia of the other eye.

2. Mechanical displacement of the lid

   A. Inflammation

      i) Trachoma—thick, heavy lid

      ii) Chalazion or hordeolum

      iii) Elephantiasis

      iv) Chronic conjunctivitis—conjunctival thickening.

      v) Traumatic or infectious edema involving the lid.

B. Tumors, especially fibromas or lipomas.

C. Scar tissue because of burns, physical trauma, and lacerations may bind the lid down.

D. Tumors of lacrimal gland—S-shaped lid.

3. Dermachalasis (ptosis adiposa, baggy lids, "puffs")—senile atrophy of the lid skin.

4. Blepharochalasis—Rare condition occurring in young individuals, characterized by recurrent bouts of inflammatory lid edema with subsequent stretching of the skin.

5. The oriental lid—The palpebral fissure is narrower than normal and upper lid rarely has a furrow; hence, the fold usually hangs down to or over the lid margin.

6. Duane syndrome (retraction syndrome).

7. Blepharospasm—eyebrow lower than normal.

AGE SPECIFIC EXOPHTHALMOS

= Most important

1. *Age*

   A. *Newborn—*

      1. Orbital sepsis

      2. Orbital neoplasm

   B. *Neonatal—*osteomyelitis of the maxilla

   C. *Early childhood* (up to 1 year of age) :

      1. Dermoid

      2. Hemangioma

      3. Dermolipoma

      4. Histiocytosis X including Hand-Schuller-Christian disease.

      5. Orbital extension of retinoblastoma.

   D. *One to five years —*

      1. Dermoid

      2. Metastatic neuroblastoma

3. Rhabdomyosarcoma

4. Epithelial cyst, such as sebaceous cyst and epithelial inclusion cyst.

5. Glioma of optic nerve

6. Sphenoid wing meningioma

7. Orbital extension of retinoblastoma

8. Fibrous dysplasia (Albright syndrome)

9. Metastatic embryonal sarcoma

* 10. Hemangioma

E. *Five to ten years —*

1. Pseudotuomor

2. Orbital extension of retinoblastoma

3. Malignant lymphomas and leukemias

* 4. Dermoid

* 5. Hemangioma

6. Meningioma

7. Fibrous dysplasia (Albright syndrome)

8. Rhabdomyosarcoma

9. Orbital hematoma

10. Glioma of optic nerve

F. *Ten to thirty years —*

* 1. Pseudotumor

2. Mucocele

3. Meningioma

* 4. Thyroid ophthalmopathy

5. Lacrimal gland tumor

6. Dermoid

7. Hemangioma

8. Peripheral nerve tumors

9. Undifferentiated sarcomas

10. Osteoma

11. Fibrous dysplasia (Albright syndrome)

12. Rhabdomyosarcoma

13. Glioma of optic nerve

G. *Thirty to fifty years* —

* 1. Pseudotumor

2. Mucocele

3. Malignant lymphomas and leukemias

4. Hemangioma

* 5. Endocrine ophthalmopathy

6. Lacrimal gland tumors

7. Rhinogenic carcinoma

8. Malignant melanoma

9. Osteosarcoma

10. Fibrosarcoma

11. Metastatic carcinoma

12. Meningioma

13. Dermoid

H. *Fifty to seventy years* —

* 1. Pseudotumor

* 2. Mucocele

* 3. Malignant lymphomas and leukemias

4. Dermoid

5. Carcinoma of palpebral or epibulbar origin

* 6. Meningioma

7. Endocrine ophthalmopathy

8. Lacrimal gland tumor

9. Osteosarcoma

10. Fibrosarcoma

11. Undifferentiated sarcoma

12. Metastatic carcinoma

13. Osteoma

14. Fibrous dysplasia (Albright syndrome)

15. Neurofibroma

16. Hemangioma

I. *More than seventy years —*

1. Melanoma

2. Pseudotumor

3. Lymphoma

4. Metastatic tumor

5. Basal cell carcinoma

6. Mucocele

NAMED SIGNS, SYNDROMES AND TESTS

1. *Adie's Pupil (Tonic Pupil)* : Somewhat resembles Argyl Robertson (AR) Pupil but of unknown aetiology, not associated with syphils, occurs in young woman, is often unilateral and associated with absent knee jerks. Pupil is slightly dilated and always larger than its fellow (whereas AR Pupil is always smaller) and reaction to light is slight and it is sluggish to coverge and is unduly sustained. It dilates with atropine (whereas AR does not).

2. *Albinism :* Hereditary condition of pigment development throughout body. It is divided into ocular (subdivided on basis of tyrosinase test), oculo-cutaneous and cutaneous forms. In first variety, iris looks pink and patient suffer from dazzling. Nystagmus, photophobia, defective vision usually present and occasionally strabismus : Ophthalmoscopy shows retinal and choroidal vessels with great clarity separated by glistening white spaces with shining sclera in between. Partial albinism is common (depigmented choroid and retina and irides being blue or macula is pigmented). Treatment is use of tinted glasses for protection against glare.

3. *Amaurosis :* Complete loss of sight in one or both eyes in the absence of ophthalmoscopic or other marked objective signs.

4. *Amblyopia :* Partial loss of vision.

5. *Amblyoscope :* (Synoptophore or orthoptoscope) : used to measure angle of the squint.

6. *Ametropia :* Errors of refraction (eg Myopia, Hypermetropia) in contrast to emmetropia (normal condition).

7. *Angioid streaks :* Dark brown or pigmented streaks, anastomosing with each other, mistaken for blood vessels, are sometimes seen of ophthalmoscopical. Differ from any normal set of blood vessels, are usually situated near the disc, at a deper level than the retinal vessels and very irregular in contour. They result due to changes in the elastic tissue of Bruch's membrane and may be associated with Pseudo-xanthoma elasticum. Vascular and degenerative choroidal lesions elsewhere in the fundus, particularly at the macula, are common developments.

8. *Ankyloblepharon :* Adhesion of the margins of the two eyelids. Treatment depends on amount. If very extensive, operation is contraindicated.

9. *Annomaloscope (Nagel's) :* Used to detect colour blindness.

10. *Aperts disease :* Acrocephaly associated with syndactylism.

11. *Arcus senilis :* Lipoid infiltration of the cornea in old people, commencing as a crescenteric grey line concentric with upper and lower corneal margins, thicker above and thin below, is formed completely around the cornea. It is separated from limbus by a line of normal cornea, sharply defined on the peripheral side. It is never more than 1 mm broad and does not affect vision or corneal vitality.

12. *Arcus juvenilis :* Similar to above but appears before the age of forty, occasionally found in old sclerosing keratitis but in this opacity is usually localized to one part of cornea and extends further towards the centre.

13. *Argyll Robertson pupil :* Spinal miosis, not reacting to light but contraction on convergence is retained. It is invariably caused by syphilitic lesion in tectum.

14. *Argyrosis :* Staining of conjunctiva as deep brown from prolonged application of silver salts (nitrate, proteinate etc.) for treatment of chronic conjunctivitis and especially trachoma.

15. *Asthenopia (accommodative or eye strain) :* Eyeache, burning in eyes and then feel dry so that blinking and lacrimation are more frequent. Results due to prolonged close work especially in the evening by artificial illumination. There may be hyperemic lids edges and frontal headache.

16. *Basedow's disease :* Grave's disease or Exophthalmic Goitre or Thyrotoxic exophthalmos

17. *Batten-Mayou Disease :* Maculo-cerebral familial degeneration, may be a delayed or juvenile form of Tay Sachs disease. It occurs in Jewish children commencing at a later age, usually six or eight years. Defective vision, central scotoma, weak intellect, convulsions and spasticity.

    Ophthalmoscopically-pale discs with small vessels, yellowish-grey spots and granular pigmentation over macula, **Pepper and Salt type pigmentation** over retina but a cherry-red spot never develops.

18. *Behcet's Disease :* A purulent uveitis with hypopyon is associated with recurrent genital conjunctival or oral aphthae. There may be neurological and articular manifestations. Seen particularly in young adults and recurs periodically and persistently in attacks of extreme severity so that eventually the vision is seriously affected or lost. The infection is probably viral but not specific treatment is available. Systemic steroids or immuno suppression are of help.

19. *Bell's phenomenon :* On closing the lids, as in sleep, the eyes generally turn upwards and outwards. The same movement occurs in attempted closure in VII nerve palsy.

20. *Benedict's syndrome :* If red nucleus is involved, tremor and jerky movements occur in the contralateral side of the body; this condition combined with ipsilateral III nerve paralysis.

21. *Berlin's Oedema :* (Commotio retinae) : Is a paralysis as a result of a blow on the eye. A milky white cloudiness due to oedema appears over a considerable area at the posterior pole. Some times, it disappears within a few days or in some, central vision gradually diminishes due to pigmentary deposits at the macula.

22. *Best's disease :* Vitelliform dystrophy of the fovea characterized by a sharply delineated, usually bilateral orange-yellow disc in the foveal disc resembling the **yolk of a fried egg**. Visual acquity remains good while neuroepithelium is unaffected. Serious loss of vision occurs after transition to an irregular pigmented lesion, after the egg has become scrambled or after haemorrhages. This leads to a polymorphous foveal dystrophy. Homogenous viscous material is present in pigment epithelium having vitelliform disc. Except central scotoma, visual fields are normal. EOG is pathological while dark adaptation and EFG are normal.

23. *Bitot's spots :* Small triangular white patches on the outer and inner sides of the cornea covered by a material dried form which is not wetted by the tears and are due to horny epithelium cast off into the conjunctival sac and accumulates in lower by. It occurs in vitamin A deficiency.

24. *Bjerrum's scotoma :* Area of relative defect in field of vision which can be frequently traced in direct continuity with the blind spot occurring in chronic simple glaucoma.

25. *Blaskowicz operation :* For ptosis in which the levator muscle is shortened by an approach from the conjunctival surface.

26. *Blepharophimosis :* Palpebral fissure appears to be contracted at the outer canthus. Outer angle is normal, but is obscured by a vertical fold of skin formed by eczematous contraction of skin following prolonged epiphore and blepharospasm (epicanthus lateralis). It requires no treatment, disappearing spontaneously or in some cases canthoplasty is done.

27. *Bourneville's disease :* (Tuberous sclerosis) Occurring in young individuals associated with nodular lesions in the CNS and skin, particularly on the face (adenoma sebacium) and retina especially near the optic nerve head. The cerebral lesions frequently lead to epilepsy and mental deficiency.

28. *Bowen's intraepithelial epithelioma :* Occurs when epitheliomata spread over the surface and into the fornices rarely penetrating the globe. They must be removed or the base being cauterized by diathermy. The diagnosis is microscopically confirmed.

29. *Bruch's membrane :* Or lamina vitrea, covering the inner side of choroid.

30. *Buerger's disease :* (Thromboangitis obliterans,) Sometimes occlusion of retinal arteries occurs resulting in the appearance of multiple retinal emboli.

31. *Buphthalmos :* Infantile or congenital glaucoma due to a failure of deve lopment of tissues in the region of angle of ant. chamber. Iris may not be completely separated from cornea and canal of Schlemm is deficient or absent.

32. ***Burrow's operation :*** for Entropion.

33. ***Campimetry :*** Field charting of central and paracentral areas

34. ***Canal of Schlemm :*** A circular venous sinus in the inner layer of sclera, bounded, posteriorly by iris root and ciliary body and anteriorly by cornea sclera. It is sometimes broken up into more than one lumen. It is important for drainage of aqueous humour.

35. ***Cataract :***

* *Black cataract or cataracta brunescens :* Occurring in senile nuclear sclerosis of lens and is due to deposition of melanins derived from the amino acids in lens.

* *Blue-dot cataract or cataract coerulea :* Small multiple opaque spots scattered all over lens, appearing as tiny blue dots on slit-lamp examination. A type of Punctate, cataract, Bread-crumbs cataract in complicated or infected cataract.

* *Hard cataract :* Occurring in elderly, due to slow sclerosis.

* *Morgagnian idiocy cataract :* Punctate subcapsular cataract.

* *Morgagnian :* Milky liquefied cortex with brown mass nuclear limited by a semicircular line; a hypermature cataract.

* *Oil drop Cataract :* in galactosemia, first lamellar cataract and then total.

* *Rossette-shaped cataract :* in injuries, usually occurs in posterior cortex, sometimes in the anterior or both.

* *Snowflakes cataract :* In Diabetes mellitus.

* *Soft cataract :* in young lens or in the cortex of adult.

* *Spindle shaped :* Or axial or coralliform or fusiform occurring as antero posterior spindle shaped opacity. A type of developmental cataract.

* *Spokes of wheel type :* in zonular cataract.

* *Sunflower cataract :* In Wilson's disease due to deposition of brilliant golden green sheen aggregated in radiating formations like the petals of a flower.

36. ***Caterpillar hairs :*** May penetrate the eye exciting a severe iridocyclitis. Characterized by formation of granulomatous nodules (Ophthalmia nodosa)

37. *Chalcosis :* Retention of copper foreign body in the eye.

38. *Chemosis :* Oedema of conjunctiva due to acute inflammations, in cases of obstruction to the circulation or abnormal blood conditions.

39. *Chromatopsia :* Coloured vision occurs in after cataract extraction (erythropsia or red vision), resolution of optic neuritis haemorrhage, snow blindness or sometimes in normal people (black print).

40. *Coats disease :* Exudative retinopathy of coats seen usually in boys, otherwise apparently normal. May be a manifestation of Battered baby syndrome. There is usually a large raised yellowish white area or several smaller areas posterior to the vessels, detachment of retina, cataract or glaucoma may occur. Haemorrhage in between retina and choroid or in deep layers of retina may occur. A similiar picture seen in angiomatosis, or in older patients. No treatment is effective.

41. *Colloid bodies :* In Tay's choroiditis —yellowish white spots in macular region due to peculiar hyaline excrescences on choroid surface.

42. *Coloboma :* One of the commonest congenital malformation in which tissues of uvea or associated retinal tissues or their prolongation associated retinal tissues or their prolongation into back of iris are badly developed.

43. *Commotio retinae :* See Berlin's oedema.

44. *Conjunctiva :*

  Pinguecula—Triangular patch on the conjunctiva in elderly especially those exposed to sunlight, dust, wind etc. occurs near limbus in the palpebral aperture, apex of triangle being away from cornea.

  Pterygium—A degenerative condition of subconjunctival tissues proliferating as vascularized granulation tissue to invade cornea destroying superficial layers of stroma and Bowman's membrane.

45. *Conjunctivitis, Beal's :* Acute conjunctivitis due to adenoviruses, may occur in epidemics may rarely cause superficial punctate keratitis, has self-limiting course.

46. *Conjunctivitis, New Castle :* Caused by Newcastle virus derived from contact with diseased fowls, indistinguishable from pharyngo-conjunctival fever (by adenovirus).

47. *Conus :* Slightly ectatic coloboma of optic disc.

48. *Corectopia :* inward displacement of pupil.

49. *Cornea :*

    Leucoma : A very dense and white corneal scar.

    Nebula : Slight thin corneal opacity.

50. *Cover test :* For diagnosis of heterophoria or squint. When one eye is covered, lateral deviation occurs in it and on removing screen, it goes to the original position.

51. *Cryptophthalmos :* A rare condition in which skin passes continuously from the brow over the eye to the cheek associated with abnormalities of the eye and often of the orbit.

52. *Descemetocele or keratocele :* Herniation of descemet's membrane through corneal ulcer as a transparent vesicle.

53. *Deuteranopia :* Green vision is defective.

54. *Devic's disease :* Neuromyelitis optica. Bilateral optic neuritis (precedes) with myelitis, with sudden onset and one eye may be affected before complete amaurosis supervenes rapidly, central scotoma, pain on moving the eyes and swelling of disc may be seen. May pass off spontaneously.

55. *Diktyoma :* Growths (malignant epithelioma) resembling embryonic retina.

56. *Distichiasis :* Rare condition in which there is extra posterior row of cilia, occasionally in all 4 lids, occupying the position of meibomian glands. These lashes may irritate cornea.

57. *Duane's retraction syndrome :* Common congenital defect due to fibrosis of lateral rectus or a contraction of lateral and medial rectus. There is defective or absent lateral deviation. On adduction, there is retraction of globe and narrowing of palpebral tissue while on abduction, there is slight exophthalmos.

58. *Eale's disease :* (Periphlebitis Retinae)—A relatively common disease of obscure aetiology (may be tubercular or septic) characterized by repeated vitreous haemorrhages (from retinal veins) occurs typically in apparently healthy young adults (usually males). It attacks

both eyes in succession and to recur, reabsorption of haemorrhages occur in early attacks but later on it persists and dense vitreous opacities and proliferative retinopathy are serious complications. Treatment is directed to cause. Other methods used are rest, a prolonged course of steroids, diathermy or light coagulation (in localized periphlebitis).

59. *Elliot's trephining :* An operation for simple glaucoma by making an-excision hole in cornea, sclera, and iris.

60. *Elschnig's pearls :* Sometimes subcapsular cells proliferate and instead of forming lens fibres, develop into large balloon-like cells which sometimes fill the pupillary aperture, (forming after or secondary cataract).

61. *Erythropsia :* Red vision occurs particularly after cataract extraction.

62. *Eversbusch's technique :* An operative technique for ptosis (to cut through skin to shorten levator muscle).

63. *Farnsworth-Munsell Test :* It represents hue discrimination by an error score, the greater the score, the poorer the colour vision.

64. *Fasanella-Servant operation :* For cases of minimal ptosis (1.5-2.0 mm) with some function of the levator.

65. *Flavone :* (Vitamin P) From citrous fruits; maintenance of health of capillaries and deficiency leads to haemorrhagic condition.

66. *Foster-Kennedy Syndrome :* Pressure atrophy of optic nerve on the side of the lesion due to direct pressure (usually from frontal meningioma or pituitary tumor) and a papilloedema on the other side due to generalized pressure.

67. *Fovea centralis :* A depression or pit, containing only cones present on the posterior pole of eye situated about **3 mm** to temporal side of optic disc.

68. *Foville Syndrome :* VI nerve palsy is replaced by a loss of conjugate movements to the same side.

69. *Friedreich's disease :* Hereditary ataxia with optic atrophy and rarely paralyses of the ocular muscles. Nystagmoid jerkings present on voluntary movements but visual symptoms are absent.

70. *Fuch's endothelial dystrophy :* Endothelial Corneal dystrophy seen in elderly (particularly females) begins with fine changes in endothelium (detected by slit lamp resulting in hyaline nodules on Descemet's membrane and eventually atrophy of underlying endothelial cells (Corneal guttate).

This is followed by epithelial dystrophy oedema, vesicles formation, opacities and insensitiviity. Blindness results. Treatment is difficult and corneal grafting sometimes ineffective.

71. *Fuchs's fleck :* In Myopic-choroido-retinal atrophy, choroidal thrombosis giving rise to sudden formation of circular claret-coloured or black spot at the fovea which persists.

72. *Fuchs's heterochromic iridocyclitis :* Low grade chronic cyclitis, resulting in lightening of the colour of the affected iris and the presence of a few keratic precipitates on the cornea; the later distinguish the condition from congenital heterochromia. Iris becomes atrophic, loses markings and readily transilluminates in circumscribed areas and a cataract frequently develops. There may be disturbed sympathetic nerve supply. Cataract has good operative prognosis but secondary glaucoma may develop.

73. *Fundus flavimaculatus :* A flecked bilateral retinal dystrophy appearing in III or IV decade. White or yellowish white deep retinal flecks resembling fish tails with fuzzy or medium-sharp outlines are seen with ophthalmoscopy. Macular effects are seen in 50% cases when central vision falls. EOG is mostly pathological indicating a diffuse retinal pigment epithelial involvement ERG and dark adoptation are normal.

74. *Von Graefe's sign :* In exophthalmic goitre, lid follows tardily or not at all.

75. *Grave's disease :* (Exophthalmic goitre or Basedow's disease) characterized by tachycardia, tremors and a raised BMR. Exophthalmos is initially unilateral and later on becomes bilateral. Signs in eye present are —*Dalrymple's sign* (unnatural degree of separation between margins of two lids), *Mobius sign* (imperfect power of convergence). Ophthalmoscopically, veins and arteries are dilated. Recovery follows control of thyrotoxic condition.

76. **Groenouw's nodular corneal dystrophy :** Of dominant heredity, granular opacities which later on coalesce into various irregular shapes.

77. **Hand Schuller Christian disease :** A type of lipodystrophy. In eye there is deposition of lipids—diabetic exophthalmic dysostosis.

78. **Harada's disease :** A disease of unknown cause (may be viral) characterized by exudative detachment of retina and choroiditis.

79. **Heerfordt's disease (Uveoparotitis) :** Bilateral involvement of entire uveal tract, parotid glands and frequently the cranial nerves, occurring in 10-30 years of age with prodromal symptoms of malaise and fever, sometimes with erythema nodosum. Half cases develop granulomatous iridocyclitis with nodules on iris, half with painful parotid swelling (like mumps) and then diplopia due to paralysis of ocular motor nerves or VII nerve palsy. It is a self limiting disease although iridocyclitis may cause permanent visual damage, parotid swelling last for 6 weeks to 2 years but also subside. The condition is probably related to sarcoidosis.

80. **Herxheimer reaction :** Acute plastic iritis occurring 24-48 hours after the first therapeutic dose of arsenic or penicillin, probably due to flooding of the system with treponemal toxins.

81. **Hess screen :** To measure the degree of deviation, especially if torsional and particularly to measure any progressive increase.

82. **Hess's operation for ptosis :** It is the simplest procedure when both muscles are paralysed:

83. **von Hippal Lindau Disease :** (Angiomatosis of Retina) A rare familial disease, occurs in III or IV decades more frequently in males. The cerebellum, medulla, spinal cord, kidneys and adrenals are precede a fatal cerebellar lesion by 10-15 years. Ophthalmoscopic appearances show most commonly a great tortuosity and dilatation of vessels together with presence of aneurysms (balloon like or small and miliary). Slowly exudates are deposited (resembling exudative retinopathy of coats). A retinal detachment may occur. Treatment is unsatisfactory but in early cases diathermic destruction or light coagulation of localized aneurysm shows beneficial effect or alternatively, the application of conizing radiation.

84. *Holmgren's Wool test :* Test for colour vision by using a selection of skins of coloured wools.

85. *Horner's syndrome :* Loss of sympathetic function on one side causing miosis, a narrowed palpebral fissure, slight enophthalmos (due to loss of tone of Muller's muscles), sometimes with unilateral absence of sweating.

86. *Hutchinson's pupil :* In concussion injuries of brain causing first contraction of ipsilateral pupil and later on dilatation (when intracranial pressure increases) and does not react to light. If pressure still increases, a similar phenomenon occurs to other pupil.

87. *Jaesche-Arlt operation :* For cicatrical entropion.

88. *"Jaw-winking" synkinesis of Marcus Gunn :* One levator palpebrae is thrown into spasm during eating and sometimes on reading aloud. There is also slight ptosis.

89. *Junius-Kuhnt's disease :* Disciform degeneration at the macula where in early stage pigment epithelium becomes separated from Bruch's membrane, and blood vessels grow into this space from chorio-capillaries, Fluorescein angiography can detect detachment of pigment epithelium and abnormal blood vessels.

90. *Kayser-Fleischer ring :* Deposit of copper forming a pigmented ring of grey-green or golden-brown colour round the periphery of the cornea in the region of Descemet's membrane and deeper layers of the stroma. Seen in hepatolenticular degeneration (Wilson's disease).

91. *Koeppe's nodules :* Minute translucent nodules appearing on the surface of iris especially at the pupillary border in exudative type of iritis (allergic in nature) e.g in sarcoidosis (Benign Lymphogranuloma).

92. **Kronlein's operation :** Lateral orbitotomy for exploration of orbital tumours.

93. *Langrange's operation :* Ordinary iridectomy done in operation for simple glaucoma.

94. *Laurence-Moon-Biedl Syndrome :* Obesity, mental defect, hypogenigenitalism and polydactyly along with pigmentary retinal dystrophy (retinitis pigmentosa).

95. **Leber cells :** Large multinucleated cells tend to be found with necrosis in follicles (formed by lymphocytes) found in trachoma.

96. **Leber's disease :** (The Amaurosis of Leber) : Pigmentary retinitis with congenital amaurosis in early infancy characterized by bilateral blindness, coarse nystagmus, some retention of pupillary reflexes and pigmentary degeneration of fundii. It is autosomal recessive. Initially there is pepper and salt type of fundus and later on bone-corpuscular form of pigmentary dystrophy develops. Optic disc becomes pale, retinal vessels attenuated and macula affected. ERG is absent and EOG defective.

97. *Little's disease (Congenital spastic diplegia) :* A bilateral spastic paralysis present from birth of degenerative cerebral process of obscure aetiology. With it, there is optic atrophy, retinal degeneration, cataract, squint and internuclear palsies.

98. *Maddox Rod test :* Simplest (next to cover test) to detect heterophoria or latent strabismus.

99. *Maddox wing test :* To test deviation in near vision.

100. *Marcus Gunn Pupil :* An afferent pupillary defect may be an earliest indication of optic nerve disease.

101. *Marcus Gunn Synkinesis :* One levator palpebrae is thrown into spasm during eating and sometimes on reading aloud. There is also slight ptosis.

102. *Marie Strumpell's disease :* (ankylosing spondylitis)—Causes in eye and acute recurrent iridocyclitis.

103. *Meibomian cyst (Chalazion Tarsal Cyst) :* It is not a cyst but chronic inflammatory granuloma of a meibomian gland. They are often multiple, occurring commonly in adults. If lid is everted, there is red or purple over the nodule and in later stages gray or yellow (hordeolum internum), may convert into a jelly like mass. Complete spontaneous resolution rarely occurs.

104. *Meibomian (tarsal) glands :* Developed schaceous glands, consisting of nearly straight tubes, directed vertically, 20-30 in numbers in each lid, each opening by a single duct on the lid margin.

105. *Mikulicz's syndrome* : Characterized by symmetrical enlargement of the lacrimal and salivary glands. The aetiology varies but swelling is usually of lymphomatous nature. Both parotid and lacrimal glands are enlarged in uveoparotid inflammation.

106. *Millard-Gubler's syndrome* : In the lower part of pontine lesion, paralysis of lateral rectus with a contralateral hemiplegia and an ipsilateral facial palsy occurs.

107. *Miners' nystagmus* : Rotatory and very rapid nystagmus in workers of coal mines, may be also associated with defective vision (worse at night), headache, giddiness, photophobia, dancing of lights and movements of objects. In dim light where vision is carried out almost entirely by rods, vision is greatest 10-15 outside fovea.

108. *Moll's glands* : Sweat glands near the edge of lids which are unusually large and situated immediately behind the hair follicles and their ducts open into the ducts of Zeis' glands or into the hair follicles.

109. *Moll's cysts* : Small clear cysts frequently occurring among the lashes in old people due to the retention of secretion of Moll's glands. They disappear if the anterior wall is snipped off.

110. *Mongolian idiocy Cataract* : Puncate subcapsular cataract in Mongols.

111. *Morgagnian cataract* : A hypermature cataract in which cortex becomes fluid and nucleus sink to the bottom of the lens.

112. *Muller's fibres* : Better developed vertical cells in nerve fibre layer (innermost) part of retina acting as a support and have nutritive function.

113. *Motais's operation* : For ptosis in which the central third of the tendon of the superior rectus is transplanted to the upper border of tarsal plate through a subconjunctival approach.

114. *Mustard gas* : Dichloroethyl sulphide producing ocular symptoms (conjunctival congestion, stippled cornea of "Orange-skin" cornea with functional blephrospasm and delayed keratitis after a latent period of 6-8 hours.

115. *Nagel's Anomalscope* : Instrument to detect defects of colour vision.

116. *New Castle's conjunctivitis :* Caused by Newcastle virus derived from contact with diseases fowls indistinguishable from pharyngoconjunctival fever (by adenovirus).

117. *Niemann Pick disease :* (Lipid Histiocytosis) Characterized by widespread changes of lipid degeneration, the hepatosplenomegaly, conjugate gaze palsies and retinal changes as found in Tay Sachs disease (e.g. a cherry red circular spot at fovea, optic atrophy etc.) occurs.

118. *Oculoglandular syndrome :* Perinaud's oculo glandular syndrome characterized by follicular conjunctivitis, preauricular (or submaxillary) lymphadenopathy. The cause varies (e.g. leptothrix, other fungi or LGV etc.)

119. *Ophthalmometer (Keratometer) :* To measure astigmatism of anterior surface of cornea at two points about 1.25 mm on either side of its centre.

120. *Orthoptoscope (Synoptophore or amblyoscope) :* To measure angle of the deviation.

121. *Perinaud's syndrome :* See oculoglandular syndrome above.

122. *Photometer (or adaptometers) :* To measure light sense or dark adaptation.

123. *Placido's keratoscopic disc :* To assess corneal surface.

124. *Preziosi's operation :* For open angle glaucoma in which a fistulous track is made into angle of anterior chamber underneath a conjunctival flap by an electro cautery.

125. *Pseudocornea :* Contraction of the bands of fibrous tissue of prolapsed iris tends to flatten the anterior chamber underneath a conjunctival flap by an electro cautery.

126. *Pseudoglioma :* A subacute form of uveitis in children which takes a plastic course characterized by the exuberent development of fibrous tissue of cyclitic origin. It gives white reflex in pupil (amaurotic cat's eye).

127. *Pseudo inflammatory foveal dystrophy of Sorsby :* Rare inherited dystrophy characterized by bilateral inflammatory signs in the posterior pole Haemorrhages, exudates, oedema and pigmentary proliferation occur. States in age of 30-50. Later on choroidal atrophy develops. Histologically represents degeneration of elastic layer of Bruch's membrane and a choroidal atrophy.

128. *Pseudo-neuritis :* A condition occurring in hyper metropic eyes when lamina is small and nerve fibres are heaped up as they. Debouch upon the retina Ophthalmoscopic appearance of swelling and blurred margins is largely due to reflexes. Swelling is less than 2 dioptes and there is no venous engorgement, oedema or exudates and blind spot is not enlarged.

129. *Purtscher's traumatic angiopathic retinopathy :* After fractures of long bones, multiple fat emboli in the retina may cause haemorrhages, and the appearance of large irregular white areas.

130. *Raynaud's disease blindness :* Spasmodic occlusion of central retinal artery in Raynaud's disease.

131. *von Recklinghausen's disease* : Elephantiasis neuromatodes, plexiform neuroma, neurofibromatosis): Affect lids and orbit (Swollen lid, temporal region affection, hypertrophied nerves due to hyperplasia of endo and perineum. Sometimes ciliary nerve affection, true glioma of optic nerve, buphthalmos may result. Choroid and ciliary body may become thickened by layers of dense fibrous tissue derived probably from cells of sheaths of Schwann. Laminated ovoid bodies resembling Pacchionian corpuscles also occur. Operative measures are seldom satisfactoy.

132. *Refractometry :* Basal on principle of indirect ophthalmoscopy to detect and measure degree of ametropia.

133. *Reis-Buckler's corneal dystrophy :* This arises in the region of Bowman's membranes, which eventually is extensively replaced by a cellular connective tissue containing collagen as well as fibrillar or granular material. The epithelium over this connective tissue shows derangement of cell layers, oedema and degeneration. The cornea shows irregular dense grey sub-epithelial opacities arranged in fishnet pattern.

134. *Reiter's disease :* Characterized by a severe purulent conjunctivitis sometimes a uveitis in association with urethritis and polyarthritis.

135. *Roenne's step :* Sectorial field defects with shortly defined horizontal edge in the upper and sometimes lower nasal fields in chronic simple glaucoma.

136. *Rubeosis Iridis :* In long standing diabetes mellitus or in thrombosis of retinal veins neovascularization in iris with signs of iritis and secondary glaucoma. Treatment is iridencleisis or partial destruction of ciliary body with diathermy or cryosurgery.

137. *Saemisch Section :* An operation, despite its name, devised by Guthrie to cut out corneal ulcer.

138. *Salzmann's corneal dystrophy :* A nodular dystrophy of cornea characterized by bluish-white nodules appearing in the superficial layers of stroma and Bowman's membrane occurring in persons with previous corneal disease. It tends to be slowly progressive and treated by lamellar keratoplasty.

139. *Scheie's operation :* Cauterization of sclera with a peripheral iridectomy to treat simple glaucoma.

140. *Schilder's disease:* Diffuse sclerosis (demyelination of entire white matter of cerebrum) occurring in young people. Ocular symptoms (Blindness due to destruction of optic radiation, optic neuritis of retrobulbar neuritis, ocular motor palsies and nystagmus) are early.

141. *Schlemm's Canal :* In chronic simple glaucoma sickle shaped extension of blind spot above and below or both with concavity of sickle directed towards the fixation point.

142. *Shadow tests :* (Retinoscopy or skiascopy) A most practical method to estimate condition of refraction objectively.

143. *Sjogren's syndrome :* Kerato-conjunctivitis sicca associated with polyarthritis. An autoimmune disease occurring in women after menopause characterized by dryness of eye (conjunctiva and cornea), fibrotic lacrimal gland and salivary glands.

144. *Sommerring's ring :* New lens fibres formed from anterior capsule (after cataract operation) which enclosed between two layers of capsule, form a dense ring behind the iris.

145. *Stallard's operation :* A flap sclerotomy done for the treatment of chronic simple glaucoma.

146. *Stargardt's disease :* A recessively progressive tapeto-retinal dystrophy of the central retina develops between 8-14 years of age. A *beaten-bronze atrophy* is seen in foveal region in late stages.

In final stages, posterior pole shows an extensive chorioretinal atrophy with poor vision. Dark adaptation, ERG and EOG are subnormal while the visual fields may become slightly restricted. Fluorescein angiography shows defects in the pigment epithelium but there is no leakage of eye.

147. *Stenopaeic test :* (Fincham's test) to differentiate halos of closed angle glaucoma from those in early cataractous changes of lens.

148. *Stevens-Johnson's syndrome :* Conjunctivitis associated with rhinits, stomatitis, urethritis and skin eruptions.

149. *Still' disease :* In children, association of rheumatoid arthritis with plastic iridocyclitis.

150. *Sturge Weber syndrome :* Association of haemangioma of choroid, leptomeninges and glaucoma. Homonymous hemianopia or epilepsy may occur. There are calcareous deposits under cerebral cortex.

151. *Strum's conoid :* The whole bundle of rays after refraction.

152. *Strum's focal interval :* Distance between two foci of rays after refraction in horizontal and vertical planes.

153. *Tay-Sachs disease (Amaurotic Family Idiocy) :* It occurs most often in Jewish children commencing during first year of life. Several family members are affected. There is gradual blindness, muscular weakness, wasting, and mental apathy progressing to idiocy. Death follows in one of two years.

   Ophthalmoscopy resembles that of embolism of central retinal artery. There is a round brilliantly white area at macula fading off peripherally into the normal fundus. In the centre of the patch is a *cherry red circular spot* at the fovea. In later stages, there is optic atrophy which is always bilateral. There is primary lipid neuronic degeneration of whole CNS including retina.

154. *Teichopsia :* Fortification spectral i.e. In the dark field bright spots and rays of various colours are often seen, frequently arranged in zig-zags. It occurs in migraine along with scintillating scotomata of various kinds.

155. *Test types :*

* *E-test :* Examiner hold E of various shapes directed in different directions. child at a distance of 6 metres has to respond to examiner to tell the direction E. It is a test of visual acquity.

* *Photostress test :* To detect macular disease (in which the recovery time is prolonged in diseased eye by at least onethird longer than normal).

* *Snellen's test :* For acquity of distant central vision. The test types are constructed upon the standard that the average minimum visual angle is 1 minute.

156. *Tritanopes :* Colour blindness due to absence of the blue sensation. (others are prolanopes when red end of the spectrum is much less bright and Deuteranopes—When green sensation of vision is defective.

157. *Ulcer, Mooren's :* (Rodent ulcer. Ulcer serpiginous) Occurs in elderly when superficial corneal layer undergoes degeneration. There is severe persistent neurologic pain and lacrimation.

158. *Ulcer serpens :* Hypopyon. Ulcer in adults most often caused by pneumococcus, with its tendency to creep over the cornea in a serpiginous fashion.

159. *Vogt-Koyanagi syndrome :* Uveitis associated with vitiligo, poliosis and deafness. A rare condition in young adults. Iridocyclitis is chronic and associated with exudative choroiditis and detachment of retina.

160. *Vossius's ring :* In some cases, a circular ring of faint or stippled opacity is seen on the ant. surface of lens due to multitudes of brown amorphous granules of pigment lying on the capsule.

161. *Weber's syndrome :* Ipsilateral ptosis and ultimately a complete IIIrd paralysis with contralateral hemiplegia involving a facial palsy of uper motor neurone type (by a lesion at intermediate level of the cerebral peduncles, the third nucleus progressively involves).

162. *de Wecker's scissors :* Used to do iridectomy (e.g. optical iridectomy with senile cataract extraction or button hole iridectomy in closed angle type).

163. *Weil's disease* : Leptospiral infection; there is jaundice with conjunctivitis and subconjunctival haemorrhage.

164. *Wharton Jones V-Y operation* : For cicatrical ectropion.

165. *Wilson's disease* : See Kayser-Fleischer ring.

166. *Zeis's glands* : The Sebaceous follicles of lids are specially differentiated and which are apart from being larger are identical with other sebacecous glands.

167. *Zonule of Zinn (Suspensory ligament)* : Lens is held in place by bundles of strands passing from surface of ciliary body to the capsule where they join to with zonules lamellae.

MISCELLANEOUS

SUDDEN LOSS OF VISUAL ACUITY

1. Acute congestive glaucoma
2. Brain injury
3. Brain stem arteriovenous malformations
4. Following orbital operation
5. Fracture of the lesser wing of the sphenoid bone
6. Injury to the optic nerve
7. Meningeal carcinomatosis
8. Occlusion of central retinal artery
9. Optic neuritis, papillitis, retrobulbar neuritis
10. Quinine poisoning
11. Retinal detachment
12. Temporal arteritis
13. Vitreous or retinal haemorrhage
14. Wood alcohol poisoning (methyl)

FUNDUS KEY

Colour	Diagnosis
Blue	Detached retina
	Retinal veins
Red	Attached retina
	Retinal arteries
	Haemorrhage

Red with outlined blue	Retinal tears
Red with hatching filled with blue	Thin retina
Black	Retinal pigmentation
Brown	Choroid pigment through detached retina
Green	Opacities in media
Yellow	Choroidoretinal exudate

FOREIGN BODIES AND REACTIONS IN EYE

	Inert substances	Mild reaction	Local reaction
Marked reaction			
Glass	Stone	Aluminium	Iron
Plastics	Lead	Zinc	Copper or brass
Porcelain			
Gold			
Silver			
Platinum			
Tantalum			

WHO's CLASSIFICATION OF XEROSIS

XN	Night Blindness
XIA	Conjunctival xerosis
XIB	Bitot's spots
X2	Corneal Xerosis
X3B	Corneal ulceration/keratomalacia affecting more than 1/3 corneal surface
X3A	Corneal ulceration/keratomalacia of less than 1/3 corneal surface.
XS	Corneal scar due to xerophthalmia

	Indirect ophthalmoscopy	Direct ophthalmoscopy
Image	True, Inverted	Virtual, erect
Magnification	4-5 times	15 Times
Illomination	Bright	Less bright
Stereopsis	Present	Absent
Field of focus	Longer	Smaller
Accesible fundus view	Up to ora serrator	Up to equator

CONTACT LENS

Indications

For the group as a whole the order of magnitudes was as follows, in terms of indications.

I. **Optical**

1. *Myopia*—As compared to glasses, contact lenses are better because of larger image better transmission, little marginal aberration, larger field, brighter perception, avoidance of rim interference etc. In myopia contact lenses are little superior to glasses as contact lenses may affect the axial length. Before giving contact lenses the error of over-correction usual in myopia may be excluded.

2. *Astigmatism*—A corneal lens fills up the irregularities of the astigmatic surface; the irregular surface of the cornea is thus replaced by regular surface of contact lens.

3. *Presbyopia*—A hyperopia exerts less accommodation with contact lenses; minor presbyopic correction in a hyperopia can therefore be delayed for a few years with contact lenses. The reverse is true for myopia; with contact lenses, presbyopia will be precipitated in presbyopic age.

4. *Keratoconus and Irregular Astigmatism*—The mode of action while using the contact lenses is the same as in regular astigmatism. The contact lens has no effect on the basic course of the disease.

5. *Aphakia*—Contact lenses are better due to smaller magnification (8% compared with 33% in spectacles), wider field, lesser marginal aberration, absence of jack in box phenomenon, more transmission, brighter, field, lesser convergence, better chances of binocularity compared to correction by spectacles.

6. *Anisometropia and Aniseikonia*—These anomalies of refractive origin are best corrected by contact lenses which bring the image size of defective eye nearer to an emmetropic eye. This helps to establish binocularity. Vertical prism imbalance of anisometropic glasses during up and down gaze is avoided. Contact lens also provides a larger field, a brighter and clearer image due to absence of aberration.

7. *Albinism*—Contact lenses better corrects the associated ametropia. Transmission may be reduced through darker tint or painted iris lenses. There is immediate improvement in photophobia.

8. *Nystagmus*—Contact lens better corrects the associated ametropia. Transmission may reduce refractive anomaly, also decreasing the amplitude of nystagmus.

9. Hyperopia

10. Aniridia

II. **Therapeutic :** Soft lenses flush fitting shells have been found useful in the following diseases :

1. Corneal burns
2. Indolent ulcers
3. Bullous keratitis
4. Stevens Johnson syndrome
5. Neuroparalytic keratitis
6. Exposure keratitis
7. Corneal edema
8. Corneal graft
9. Pemphigus
10. Kerato-conjunctivitis Sicca
11. Descemetocoele
12. Trichiasis
13. Symblepharon (a scleral shell is given after cutting adhesions)
14. Leaking wounds
15. Small traumatic corneal wounds
16. Recurrent erosions
17. Dry eyes.

In recent years, soft lenses (2 hydroxy ethyl methylacrylate) HEMA) are gaining ground over hard lenses of polymethylmethacrylate (PMMA); the latter, however, remain superior in providing better visual activity.

III. **Cosmetic**

1. *Unsightly corneas* or eye balls can be hidden by the painted or tinted contact lens. A deformed eye with useful vision is corrected by a painted lens with clear pupil which bears the optical correction as in adherent leucoma.

   Prosthetic—Here contact lenses may be

A. Scleral when it may be used as :

(i) Prosthetic haptic with clear optic or vice-versa.

(ii) Occlusion of pupil as in complicated cataract with retinal dysfunctions or clear pupil as in aniridia.

(iii) Partial prosthetic in partial aniridia and peripheral corneal opacities.

(iv) Ptosis props

(v) Orbital prosthesis

B. Corneal-extra limbal corneal lenses for aniridia.

2. Actors : Colour of the underlying light coloured iris can be changed.

IV. Occupational

1. Temperature variation : Fogging of spectacles is avoided while shifting from cold to hot and humid temperature, as contact lenses are at same temperature as the body.

2. News Casters and television actors are enabled to avoid reflection that occurs with spectacles.

3. Sports : Contact lenses have an advantage because of better optics, lesser hazards of serious injury compared to spectacles.

V. Diagnostic

Contact lenses are used in the following instruments where they are used to neutralise cornea to pick up its potentials, or as marker.

1. *Gonioscopy.* This is to see angle, and to operate on angle in infantile glaucoma.

2. *Fundoscopy.* Has a high minus central lens neutralises the cornea so that fundus can be viewed directly. It is much more comfortable if soft lens is placed underneath.

3. *Electrodiagnostic procedure.* Electrode incorporation is used in the lens to pick potentials at the cornea. Gold, Silver or Platinum wires can be used. Scleral lens with electrode or electrode sandwiched between two soft lenses are used in electro-retinography and its finer components like early receptor and oscillation potentials.

VI. Research

Contact lens may be used in research for :

1. Stimulating accommodation with minus lenses.

2. Relaxing accommodation with minus lenses.

3. Noting the eye movements by seeing movements of reflected light from a mirror attached to the front surface of scleral lens.

4. Temperature measurements :

   (a) By implanting thermister through a haptic lens. This is a small ceramic device which created different electrical potentials with changes in temperature.

   (b) It is also done by noting changes in colour of heat-sensitive crystals laminated with in the contact lens.

5. Measurement of lid pressure through planting a transducer on the front surface of haptic lens.

6. Getting a stabilised retinal image through a scleral lens, used to neutralise small involuntary movements of the eye.

7. Study of surface tension after of lens parameters. Through a small hook on the front surface of the lens; force needed to detach, this lens from the cornea is measured.

8. Experimental studies on animals for occlusion, hemianopic effects, to stimulate or relax accommodation and protection of the eye under anaesthesia, also used as splints in corneal grafts.

Contact Lens : Contra indications

1. *Palpebral*

   1. Stye
   2. Chalazion of upper lid
   3. Trichiasis
   4. Entropion
   5. Ectropion
   6. Squamous blepharitis
   7. Ulcerative blepharitis

2. *Conjunctival*
   1. Chronic hyperaemia
   2. Acute bacterial, viral and fungal conjunctivitis
   3. Allergic conjunctivitis
   4. Vernal conjunctivitis
   5. Symblepharon
   6. Pterygium
3. *Corneal*
   1. Epithelial dystrophies
   2. Pannus formation
   3. Corneal ulcer
   4. Keratitis
4. *Paralysis of Fifth Nerve*
5. *Exophthalmos*
   The upper lid does not reach the upper limbus, so the lens is not picked-up by the lids.
6. *Other Ocular conditions*
   1. Scleritis
   2. Episcleritis
   3. Acute or chronic iritis
   4. Cyclitis
   5. Choroiditis
   6. Uncontrolled diabetes
   7. Glaucoma with bleb
7. *Non-Medical causes*
   Non medical factors which may affect the successful use of contact lenses are :
   1. Motivation
   2. Sex
   3. Complexion
   4. Type & extent of refractive error
   5. Degree, sign & site of astigmatism
   6. Corneal toricity
   7. Visual acuity without glasses

Contact lenses are :

* *Hard*—Which are now rarely used, but are indicated for high astigmatism and corneal ectasia such as keratoconus. They are generally microlenses, their edge lying well within the limbus.

* *Soft hydrophilic*—Composed of hydroxymethyl methacrylate, which retain 25-85% hydration. They are usually large in diameter and overlap the limbus.

* *Gas permeable*—With a low water content, and high oxygen permeability.

  Generally, contact lenses are removed at the end of each day, but on occasions are worn for up to seven days (intermediate wear) or for periods of up to three months (permanent wear).

Complications of contact lens

(A) **Corneal complications**

(i) *Vascularisation of the cornea*

This occurs particularly in intermittent wear, or permanent wear. It is generally seen as superficial vessels at the upper limbus, and indicates that the patient needs to have the lens changed and refitted.

(ii) *Punctate epithelial staining*

This occurs in varying distributions and generally indicates that further advice is necessary. It may occur in several situations.

* Linear staining in the lower part of the cornea, induced by trauma associated with insertion or removal.

* Central corneal staining occurs in flat, fitted lenses.

* Punctate erosions in the lower part of the cornea may result from inadequate blinking.

* Peripheral arcuate staining occurs at the rim of a lens with a thickened edge, as in the case of a high minus lens.

* Hypoxia occurs in a tightly fitted lens and gives rise to diffuse or focal staining.

(iii) *Small, sterile, corneal ulcers*

These can occur, but generally resolve. They must, of course, be investigated in usual way in the hospital clinic.

(iv) *Bacterial infection*

This results from introduction of organisms from infected lenses or lens solutions, contaminated fingers, or inadequate disinfection techniques. The patient will need admission and immediate investigation as early treatment is essential to preserve useful vision.

(v) *Acanthamoeba infection*

This is a rare condition occurring in contact lens wearers. It induces chronic ulcerative keratitis, which presents at the early stages with an epithelial deficit and stromal haze. It may mimic herpes simplex keratitis.

INTRAOCULAR LENSES

IOL Materials

* **Optics :** Most are made from polymethyl methacrylate (PMMA Perspex CQ). Index of refraction of PMMA is **1.49** and specific gravity is : **1.19** Foldable optics are made from either silicone, hydrogel, or acrylic.

* *Haptics :* most are made from PMMA, P-CQ, polypropylene, or proline.

* *Sterilization :* is by ethylene oxide gas. Lenses should be rinsed before insertion to rinse off any residual chemical.

IOL power estimation

* Crude estimate of lens power necessary to approximate emmetropia can be made by assuming an 18D IOL will restore basic refraction to plano in an emmetropic eye. If one wishes to "emmetropize" an eye then 1.25 D should be added to 18 for each diopter of hyperopia to be corrected and 1.25 D substracted from 18 per each diopter of myopia to be corrected.

* Accurate measurement of lens power necessary for desired postoperative refraction is made by obtaining ultrasonic axial length, keratometry readings, and manufacturer's estimates of postoperative AC depth and placing these measurements in various mathematical formulas or programs.

* Formulas to calculate lens powers used most frequently include Binkhorst, Sanders-Retzlaff-Fraff, and Colenbrander-Hoffer.

Common sources of errors

* Error in axial length measurement (0.1 mm error corresponds to error in final refraction of approximately 0.25 D).

* Error in keratometry readings (0.1 error in radius measurement corresponds to error in final refraction of approximately 0.50 D).

* Error in postoperative AC depth estimates (0.1 mm error corresponds to error in final refraction of approximately 0.05-0.25 D).

IOL Design

* There is a plethora of IOL designs; however, they can be categorized into posterior chamber lenses, iris supporting lenses, and anterior chamber lenses.

* Trends show that J-loop and C-loop posterior chamber lenses dominate the market. The variety of anterior chamber designs has decreased.

Small incision IOL

Advantages

* Insertable through smaller incision than conventional PMMA IOLs. Therefore, reduced incidence of incision-related complications and more rapid vision recovery (decreased astigmatism).

Disadvantages

* Shorter track record of foldable lens material compared to PMMA
* More difficult to insert than conventional PMMA IOLs

Properties of Foldable IOLs

* Silicone (Starr, AMO)

  — refractive index : 1.42 (Starr), 1.46 (AMO).

  — hydrophobic, moderately fragile.

  — IOL design : multipiece or single piece biconvex optic only (limits compressibility).

  — incision size : 4.0 mm

  — manufacturing : east molded (does not remove monomers, impurities), produces smooth optical surface-no tumbling needed.

* *Hydrogel (Alcon)*
  — refractive index : 1. 43
  — hydrophilic (may reduce tissue damage), very fragile
  — IOL design : single piece only, biconvex optic only (limits compressibility)
  — incision size : 4.0 mm
  — manufacturing : lathe cut (dehydrated state), hydrated to acquire full dimension
* *Acrylic (Ioptex, Optical Radiation Corp)*
  — refractive index : 1.48
  — hydrophobic, very elastic (temperature-dependent), not fragile (resists tearing)
  — IOL designs : multipiece or single piece, biocnvex or plano convex (more compressible)
  — Incision size : 3.0 to 4.0 (Ioptex)
  — manfufacturing : lathe cut (cryogenic), impurities removed before lathing, cyotumbling required

---

OPHTHALMIC LASERS

Principles

* Light occupies a small part of the electromagnetic specturm
  — optical portion includes visible light (between 400 and 700 nm)
  — flanking portions are infrared on the long end and ultraviolet on the short end
  — x-rays are of even shorter wavelength whereas radio and microwaves are longer.
* The word laser is an acronym for **Light Amplication by Stimulated Emission of Radiation** phase and is thus potentially powerful and easily focused.
* There are **three basic components** of a laser system :
  — a laser medium
  — an energy (for pumping) source
  — an amplification chamber or cavity with a means of releasing some of the amplified energy.

---

* Laser **medium** may be :

  — solid (e.g. neodymium supported by a Yag crystal)

  — liquid (e.g. dye laser)

  — gas (e.g. argon, krypton, CO2)

* The energy source may be :

  — an electric discharge (e.g. gas laser).

  — another laser source (e.g. dye laser).

  — an incoherent light source (e.g. solid crystal laser).

* The energy source raises the atoms of the laser medium to a higher energy state—the subsequent return to ground state is accompanied by the emmision of a photon ("light bundle") of energy.

* The continuous pumping of the medium with internal oscillation of the photons within the cavity eventually leads to a **"population inversion"** where most of the contained atoms are in a higher than ground state energy level.

* The laser cavity is bounded by mirrors, one of which is 100% reflective while the other is partially reflective (partially transparent) to the contained laser light—a portion of the photons striking this second mirror will leave the cavity as emitted laser light.

* Continuous wave laser such as argon and krypton create their effects by heating tissue (**photocoagulation**)—This depends on the absorption of light energy by pigmented tissues (containing melanin, hemoglobin, and xanthophyll) and the coversion of this energy to heat, which produces the consequent thermal effects on the target tissue.

* Pulsed lasers such as the Nd : Yag create their effect by impact and shock wave (**photodisruption**)—This effect is independent of target pigmentation.

COMPARISON OF OPHTHALMIC SUTURE MATERIALS

Suture material	Relative tensile strength	Relative holding duration	Relative tissue reaction	Ease of handling	Special knot required	Behaviour of exposed ends	Available sizes
Surgical gut or collagen							
Plain	6	1 week	4+	Fair	No	Stiff	4.0 to 6.0
Chronic	6	< 2weeks	3+	Fair	No	Stif	4.0 to 8.0
Polyglactin 910							
Braided	9	2 weeks	2+	Good	Yes	Stiff	4.0 to 9.0
Monofilament	9	2 weeks	2+	Good	Yes	Stiff	9.0 to 10.0
Polyglycolic acid	9	2 weeks	2+	Good	Yes	Stiff	9.0 to 10.0
Silk							
Virgin	7	2 months	3+	Excellent	No	Softest	8.0 to 9.0
Braided	8	2 months	3+	Good	No	Soft	4.0 to 9.0
Polyamide (Nylon)	9	6 months	1+	Fair	Yes+	Stiff & sharp	8.0 to 11.0
Polyprophylene	10	>12 months	1+	Fair	Yes	Stiff & Sharp	4.0 to 6.0

* The higher the number the greater the relative tensile strength. Strength varies with size of material : estimates apply mainly to size 8-0 sutures.

* Holding duration will vary with location and size of suture, health of patient, medications employed, etc. The time given in this table is an average of the time at which about 30% of tensile strength is lost.

* 1+ indicates least inflammatory response; 4+ greatest.

* With needles appropriate for ophthalmic use. Sizes available will vary from time-to-time.

LASERS IN COMMON USE

Argon laser blue (488 nm, ALB) and argon laser green (514 nm, ALG)

* Most commonly used laser in ophthalmology today.

* ALB and ALG: Lasers of choice for panretinal photocoagulation, direct coagulation of retinal neovascularization, some focal retinal treatments, and all anterior segment procedures.

* ALG better suited than ALB for direct treatment of microneurysms in the macula.

Krypton laser red (647 nm)

* Damage restricted to choroid and outer retina

* Treatment of choice for choroidal neovascular membranes in the macula.

* No absorption by the macular luteal pigment so that 85% of krypton energy passes into the choroid

* Little energy absorbed by hemoglobin; therefore; one can safely coagulate beneath parafoveal blood vessels.

* Intraretinal fibrosis does not occur after treatment.

* Permits treatment of choroidal neovascularization even within the foveal avascular zone.

Dye laser (577 nm to 630 nm)

* Rhodamine 6G (stimulated by high powered argon laser), which pumps dye into action.

* Can selectively target individual tissue within the eye.

* Commonly used wavelengths :

— 577 nm; excellent for photocoagulation of blood vessels and melanin, less lens scatter than argon or krypton lasers.

— 630 nm: primary absorption by melanin in choroid and RPE., haemoglobin minimal; excellent for panretinal photocoagulation with vitreous haemorrhage present.

* subretinal neovascularization may be best treated by dye laser using combined wavelengths 630 nm and 577 nm.

Neodymium Yag Laser (1064 nm)

* clinical applications
    — *Posterior capsulotomy* : Provides a noninvasive technique for cutting posterior capsule of lens after opacification develops.
    — *Iridectomy* : does not depend on pigment. therefore excellent in blue irides.
    — *Vitreous membrane* lysis; multiple sessions often required.
* spot size fixed at 50 nm.
* HeNe (helium neon) is coaxial aiming laser that is aligned slightly anterior to YAG beam.
* Optical breakdown: microexplosion generated by high power density.
* Plasma is an altered state of matter wherein electrons have been dissociated from their atoms.
* Photodisruption : laser functions by creating shock wave rather than thermal effect.
* Q-switched mode (one-billonth of a second pulse) permits shorter burst (one trillonth of a sec.)

---

* **Ocular Findings in Selected Chromosomal Syndromes**

Trisomy Syndromes	Ocular Findings
Trisomy 8	Hypertelorism, downward slanting of palpebral fissures, strabismus, blepharospasm bleopharophimosis, corneal opacities, cataract, iris heterochromia, colobomatous microphthalmia, megalocornea, retinal vessel tortuosity
Trisomy 9	Up-or downslanting of the palpebral fissure, narrow palpebral fissure, hypertelorism. Epibulbar dermoid, corneal oapcities, enophthalmos, microphthalmia.
Trisomy 13 (Patau Syndrome)	Colobomatous microphthalmia, cyclopia, cataracts, corneal opacities, glaucoma, persistent hyperplastic primary vitureous, intraocular cartilage and retinal dysplasia. Anophthalmia, microcornea, optic nerve hypoplasia epicanthus, hypertelorism

Trisomy 14	Hypo and hypertelorism, downslanting of the palpebral fissure, blepharooptosis, deep set eyes, eversion of the eyelids, Microphthalmia.
Trisomy 18 (Edwards Syndrome)	Epicanthus, hypoplastic supraorbital ridges, Corneal opacities, Congenital glaucoma, cataract, microcornea, retina pigment epithelial alteration, cyclopia, colobomatous microphthalmia, blepharoptosis, hypertelorism, strabismus
Trisomy 21 (down syndrome)	Epicanthus, upward staring of the palpebral fissure refractive errors (especially high myopia). strabismus, nystagmus, blepharitis, eyelid ectropion, keratoconius, Brushfield iris spots, glaucoma, congenital or acquired cataracts, abnormal retinal blood vessels.
Trisomy 22	Epicanthus, hypertelorism upward or downard slanting of palpebral fissure, colobomatous microphthalmia, strabismus, blepharoptosis, synophtys, cataract dislocated lenses, optic nerve hypoplasia, persistent hyperplastic primary vitrous, myopia

Monosomy syndromes   Ocular Findings

| Monosomy 21 | Epicanthus, downward slanting of the the palpebral fissures, Peters anomaly of the anterior segment cataracts, microphthalmia. |
| Monosomy 22 | Epicanthus, hypertelorism, upward slanting of the palpebral fissure, blepharoptosis |

Sex   **Ocular findings**
Determining
Chromosomal syndromes

| Turner's Syndrome | Ptosis, strasbismus, cataracts refractive errors, corneal scars, blue sclera, color blindness hypertelorism, epicanthus, antimogoloid slant, abnormalities of retinal blood vessels, nystagmus |
| Klinefelter's syndrome | Epicanthal folds, hypertelorism, upward slant of palpebral fissure, strabismus, Brushfield spots, myopia, choroidal atrophy, colobomatous microphthalmia |

2